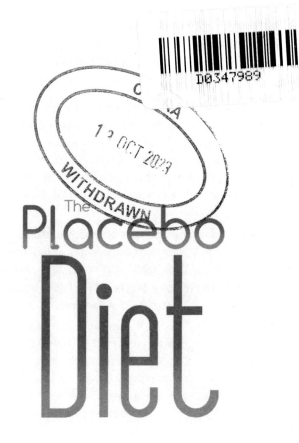

The
Placebo
Diet

The Placebo Diet

Use Your Mind
to Transform
Your Body

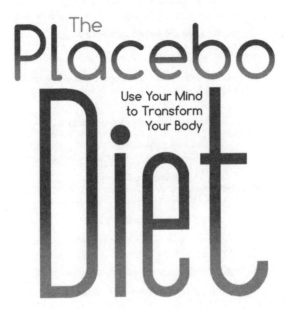

JANET THOMSON MSc

HAY HOUSE

Carlsbad, California • New York City • London • Sydney
Johannesburg • Vancouver • Hong Kong • New Delhi

First published and distributed in the United Kingdom by:
Hay House UK Ltd, Astley House, 33 Notting Hill Gate, London W1 1 3JQ
Tel: +44 (0)20 3675 2450; Fax: +44 (0)20 3675 2451; www.hayhouse.co.uk

Published and distributed in the United States of America by:
Hay House Inc., PO Box 5100, Carlsbad, CA 92018-5100
Tel: (1) 760 431 7695 or (800) 654 5126
Fax: (1) 760 431 6948 or (800) 650 5115; www.hayhouse.com

Published and distributed in Australia by:
Hay House Australia Ltd, 18/36 Ralph St, Alexandria NSW 2015
Tel: (61) 2 9669 4299; Fax: (61) 2 9669 4144; www.hayhouse.com.au

Published and distributed in the Republic of South Africa by:
Hay House SA (Pty) Ltd, PO Box 990, Witkoppen 2068
info@hayhouse.co.za; www.hayhouse.co.za

Published and distributed in India by:
Hay House Publishers India, Muskaan Complex, Plot No.3, B-2,
Vasant Kunj, New Delhi 110 070
Tel: (91) 11 4176 1620; Fax: (91) 11 4176 1630; www.hayhouse.co.in

Distributed in Canada by:
Raincoast Books, 2440 Viking Way, Richmond, B.C. V6V 1N2
Tel: (1) 604 448 7100; Fax: (1) 604 270 7161; www.raincoast.com

Text © Janet Thomson, 2016

A significant portion of this book was originally published as
Think More, Eat Less (ISBN: 978-1-84850-712-8).

The moral rights of the authors have been asserted.

The information given in this book should not be treated as a substitute
for professional medical advice; always consult a medical practitioner. Any
use of information in this book is at the reader's discretion and risk. Neither
the authors nor the publisher can be held responsible for any loss, claim or
damage arising out of the use, or misuse, of the suggestions made, the failure
to take medical advice or for any material on third party websites.
A catalogue record for this book is available from the British Library.

ISBN: 978-1-78180-665-4

Interior images: 9 Thinkstock/Sfischka; 23, 167 M.Gove/dollarphotoclub.com; 152
Thinkstock/vicvic13/kowalska-art/bagotaj; 166 Thinkstock/Amedghousse Abdellah;
Thinkstock/ttsz; all other images © Janet Thomson & Hay House UK

Printed and bound by CPI Group (UK) Ltd, Croydon, CR0 4YY

Contents

Acknowledgements

I hope that this book enlightens and inspires you. I have poured my professional heart and soul into it and dedicate it to you. If you are reading it then it is because you want to change. You want something better. I have good news: everything you need is within.

In as much as I hope that my work inspires you, this is my opportunity to say a huge thank you to those who have inspired and supported me over the last few years.

My children, Ben Ryan and Emilie, and my parents, Ken and Rita Eagle, are my inspiration for everything; they always will be. It's the kind of unconditional love that knows no bounds and has been the most constant and precious feature in my life.

One inspirational lady I have had the pleasure to get to know and work with, and who has inspired me to create programmes that help people change how they think and feel, is Dr Suhair Hassan Al Qurashi. She is president of Dar Al-Hekma University in Jeddha, Saudi Arabia. This amazing institution is dedicated to inspiring its female students to step up and believe in their own ability. Earlier this year I visited the university as a guest lecturer and taught my 'Change Your Mind' programme to over 400 faculty and staff. It was an amazing experience and the enthusiasm of the students, under Dr Suhair's leadership, knows no bounds.

If you approach this book with a fraction of the enthusiasm they embraced many of the same techniques with, then magic will happen.

In addition to my many amazing friends, there are four people, both friends and colleagues, who share my passion for helping people feel, and be, the best they can. Dr Mark Chambers has provided me with a constant supply of neurological books and papers (and no small amount of encouragement), which proved invaluable. Kevin Laye, a fellow therapist and author, and Steve McNulty, also an author and executive corporate coach, are a constant source of inspiration, and encourage me to stretch myself, professionally as part of the Growing Wellness team and personally. Special thanks also to the amazing Kay Westrap, not just for building the www.theplacebodiet.co.uk website and online programme but for being my 'business mum' and an inspiration to everyone she meets.

Thank you to the inspirational Morris Goodman, who you will meet inside this book. He is simply an amazing man.

Without wanting this to turn into an Oscars speech, I must also thank Michelle Pilley and Jo Burgess at Hay House for embracing the uniqueness of *The Placebo Diet*.

At the end of the book you will find a recommended reading list. The beautiful books you will find here have informed, inspired and enlightened me, and I encourage you to read and embrace this list.

•••••••••••••••••••••••••••••

Introduction

Welcome to the Placebo Diet. First things first – if you follow the guidelines and exercises in this book you will lose weight. That's the only reason it's called a 'diet'. However, it's unlike any diet you have ever seen before, because although there's nutrition advice and a colour-code system to make it super simple to follow, this programme is more about how to change your mind, and reprogramme your brain so that you naturally make different food choices, with no willpower required.

I have been helping people just like you lose weight for over 25 years; along the way I have learned a lot about what works and why, and even more about what doesn't work – and why. For example, I know putting yourself on a regime that means not having many of the foods you enjoy, and having to deny yourself the pleasure associated with those foods, does not work. No wonder so many people give up! If it's not something you can change permanently without feeling deprived, then it's never going to work long term. You can only sustain it as long as you can overcome your fundamental desire to feel pleasure, which ranges between a few days and a few weeks for most people.

One January a couple of years ago, I was doing a live radio phone-in answering questions about why so many diets fail. Research (commissioned by Kellogg's) had just been published in which women were asked what they thought their chances of success would be at the beginning of their diet and 70 per cent said they believed they would fail. It was around 11:30 a.m., and one caller said she had already given up yet another failed diet attempt. I asked her when she had started the diet expecting her to say a few days or maybe weeks ago but she said, 'Nine o'clock this morning!' You might laugh as you read this but that's surprisingly common.

I spent many years studying Nutrition and Exercise Science (MSc) and as a result, created my colour-code system to simplify the process of what best to eat in order to lose weight. When I ran my own health clubs I used this system with my members to great effect and each year we awarded a special prize to the achiever or slimmer of the year in each of the three clubs. The prize included a free makeover where we took the lucky winners to buy a new outfit, before getting their make-up done for a photoshoot. On one occasion the three winners were asked to go out into the store and pick the outfit they thought suited them best so we could get an idea of what they liked, before the styling began. One girl who had gone from a UK size 22/24 to a size 8/10 in 18 months came back with a size 14 black and grey dress that looked more like a quilt cover. I was astonished and said to her, 'You do realize that you are not fat anymore?' She just looked at me blankly. I could see in that moment that she was still thinking like a fat person. I knew that if she was still buying clothes with that mind-set then it was only a matter of time before everything else reverted back to exactly the same old fat-thought process. It was a powerful learning curve for me having spent years perfecting my colour-code system. I realized that without the right mental approach it was virtually worthless and that, despite a decade of studying and helping people, on many levels I knew very little about weight loss. I can tell you my professional ego took a bit of a hit as I was already a bestselling author and television 'expert', with a number-one fitness DVD. That was 12 years ago.

If someone wanted to tone their arms, I could teach them a biceps curl and explain to them exactly what was happening inside their body to that muscle and why it worked. For example, muscle is made up of fast twitch and slow twitch fibres – fast twitch ones build strength and slow twitch ones increase endurance. I could build an effective programme around this knowledge and predict the results. Clients would also be able to see their arms change shape over a few weeks, as evidence or reward for their efforts.

What I couldn't explain at the time was how thoughts work and what happens inside the brain when we think; why some people succeed and others don't. Also – there's the small matter of not being able to look at your head after a few weeks and notice the brain changing shape so that you know you are on the right lines. A biceps curl works for anyone who wants to strengthen that particular muscle, but brains are a bit more individual than muscles and are not as predictable. It's our brains that determine whether or not we are going to succeed, so learning how a brain works became my number one priority.

The next day I began a relentless search for different, effective ways to help people to change their minds. This search has resulted in my attending many practical therapeutic and coaching courses (many of which I now teach) which you will learn more about throughout the book. From all of these I have compiled the very best mind-changing exercises and adapted them to include some of my own unique techniques so that you can change your mind and transform your body.

The most common feedback I get from my clients, whether they follow the online at-home package or come to my seminars or retreats, is, 'I can't believe I am losing weight and I am not on a diet – it just feels so natural!

. . . .

Chapter 1

How to Use This Book

The first few chapters give an overview of brain function and
how we learn, create and change habits, and, of course, the
placebo effect. Most of the concepts introduced in this section are
explained in more detail later in the book, however this section
is important as it sets the scene for the subsequent chapters,
which contain the practical exercises that will change your mind
and transform your body. Considering your brain is in charge of
all areas of your life, a user-friendly guide to how to use it might
prove more useful than you think.

The basis for this book is the exciting new advances scientists
have made in understanding how the brain works in terms of
behaviours and habits. The one thing we have become most
aware of is just how plastic the brain is, meaning it is capable of
moulding and changing. In *The Placebo Diet* I'll be teaching you
how to change your brain and transform your thoughts and
behaviours so that weight loss is a happy, inevitable consequence
of the changes, along with many other changes that you will find
at least as positive.

Throughout the book you will find a mixture of technical
information that will teach you how your brain works, interspersed

with the practical exercises. This balance of theory and practice has been carefully constructed so that some changes you can make without thinking, just by reading the book, and others you can make more deliberately by doing the exercises. This is the same for the mind element and for the nutrition element of the book where the mixture of information and practical application has been put together in an enticing cocktail.

There is a free practical journal to accompany this book on my website www.theplacebodiet.co.uk. It's extremely important, if not vital, you download this as a working document. Research has shown time and again that when you keep a journal you are more successful. It's such a simple thing to do and this one is more useful than just a blank notebook as I have given you the structure, in the form of exercises, to record the things that are most important in helping you to change.

I have done as much as I can but I cannot keep your personal journal for you. If you can't be bothered to do it then maybe stop reading right now and pick this book up again when you are ready to put the effort in. If that sounds rude, that's not my intention – but it is my intention to be brutally honest with you. A coach isn't a best friend – you already have those! Over the next few weeks, as you learn how to change and what to change, you will need to do your part. It's an interactive process, technology hasn't quite evolved to the scene in *The Matrix* where Neo needs to learn to fly a helicopter to escape so he downloads the software straight into his brain, just in time to fly away! Take responsibility for your actions. I saw this great quote on the internet this week, which sums it up perfectly. Keep it in mind:

'You are free to choose, but you are not free from the consequence of your choice.'

If you want a more practical approach to go along with the book you can also follow the 'Placebo Diet at Home' programme that you can find on the website where I personally guide you through the process using videos and guided meditations. I also run practical workshops and luxury retreats and you will find details of these on the website if you would like to build on what you learn here.

There is some scientific explanation about neurological processes in this programme, which you may not expect in a diet book. It is well known that knowledge really is power. In life coaching there's a term: 'Awareness is curative'. This means once you are aware something harms you then you are less driven to do it. When you understand how and why your brain works, and why you have become programmed to do certain things, it gives you the power to change (that's why I called my therapy business 'Power To Change.Me'). *You* really do have the power to change yourself and that doesn't just mean your weight, but anything you are not happy with.

Why Is It Called the 'Placebo' Diet?

The title, *The Placebo Diet*, is very relevant because a placebo makes you believe that something in your external world (in medical trials this would be a fake tablet or other medical process) will change something in your internal world, i.e. cause cells inside your body to heal.

There has been much discussion over whether or not the placebo effect is real, but it is an essential part of any clinical trial, as the effectiveness of the new drug has to be measured against a drug that is totally inactive. If both groups in the trial get better, then the success of the healing cannot be attributed entirely to the specific drug being tested. In most clinical trials a significant percentage of patients get better on the fake medication, i.e. the placebo, and this can vary from 30 percent to much higher.

The American Cancer Society reports on their website that, 'Scientists have recorded brain activity in response to placebo. Since many scientific tests have shown that there is a placebo effect, it's one way we know for sure that the mind and body are connected.'

The UK NHS website states, 'The placebo effect is an example of how our expectations and beliefs can cause real change in our physical bodies. It's a phenomenon that we don't completely understand but we can see it working in all kinds of ways, and all kinds of circumstances'. Whatever your viewpoint as to how it works (more about this as we go through the programme), it's now widely accepted as a very real and regular occurrence.

So what has that got to do with weight loss? The answer is – more than you think, because it tells us so much about how our brains work and, most importantly, how we can literally change our minds.

When you watch most romantic comedies such as *Bridget Jones's Diary*, or some episodes of *Sex and the City*, you will see romantic pain being soothed by a nice bowl of ice cream, or perhaps a glass (or two!) of wine. On the screen the actress appears comforted. Our mirror neurons (more about these later) pick up on this and we, too, start to associate comfort with these kinds of food and drink. We 'learn' that these foods are comforting and make powerful associations and assumptions. There's no magic chemical or ingredient in the ice cream that makes us feel good, but it works because we believe it will. This is another example of something in our external world changing our internal world, in this case changing how we feel. This is significant because, as you will learn, everything we do is to get a feeling. Imagine feeling good as a default setting, and every time you get a bad or painful feeling you choose to do or think something that makes you feel good again. It's a natural process; no one deliberately chooses to do or think the things they know will make them feel bad. Even the worst habits or patterns give us at least a moment of pleasure otherwise we wouldn't do them.

We avoid the pain of emotional distress and use food as a placebo. When certain foods make us feel happy (because we believe they will) this simply reinforces the belief that we were right. The association between that food and feeling good becomes hard-wired, so the next time we need to feel comfort we are driven to eat it again. If we associate pain with having to stop eating certain foods that we like and find comforting, our minds are naturally geared to override that signal, and to avoid the emotional deprivation associated with not eating it, we eat the food. It's a never-ending cycle.

As humans we are designed to avoid pain and achieve pleasure. It's a survival instinct because, in extreme cases, pain can mean death. It's an in-the-moment decision, in other words your brain asks, 'Will this help me avoid pain *right now*?' If the answer is, 'Yes', there's a fundamental drive to avoid whatever it is that will cause the pain in that moment. The problem is that instinct is used invariably, whether it's appropriate or not. If someone who has early stage heart disease due to body shape and size, looks at a cream cake that they perceive as tasting delicious and asks themselves, 'Will not having this cake bring me pleasure or pain?' The instant answer is, 'Not having it will bring me pain' – so to avoid that feeling they eat the cake. Totally ignoring the fact that medium and longer term it will actually bring massive pain – quite literally if they end up having a heart attack. What's more, *because they believe the cake will make them feel better – it does. That's the placebo effect.*

Doctors have known about the power of the placebo effect for decades; up until the late 1960s it was part of routine care and doctors in the US could legally prescribe placebos, and even specify what colour the sugar pill should be. All this stopped when the civil rights revolution pressed for more patient autonomy and informed consent. Currently the only available inert pill is Obecalp (placebo spelled backwards) which is a cherry-flavoured pill aimed at children.

The most important fact is that the placebo effect is based on having a belief that is so unquestioning and powerful, it can change our neurology as well as our cell biology. In terms of health, the placebo effect has been shown to evoke spontaneous, medically unexplainable healing and genuine, measurable, biological change within our cells. For the past few years I have been interested in taking this principle and exploring how we can use the placebo effect to change the cells in our brain (neurons) that generate thoughts, feelings and behaviours. Through my workshops and retreats, and through the online programme (Placebo Diet at Home), I have been using the exercises you will find here with great results. My clients have been able to reprogramme their belief systems, create new habits and behaviours and associate pleasure with them, and of course lose weight.

I am often asked if this is a form of hypnosis. Although there are many guided meditations in the Placebo Diet at Home online programme, and through some of the exercises in this book, if anything I am un-hypnotizing you. You will be able to see things more clearly and change your view or reality, replacing many of your associations with food so that a new way of eating evolves naturally and without any sense of dieting.

This means you can do the things that will genuinely bring you the most pleasure (starting with weight loss and more vitality) and generate 'happy' brain chemicals that make you feel good in the moment and longer term. It's a win:win process.

The main aim of the book is to change how you think and feel about food – but you may well get a lot more than you bargained for – and start feeling good about many other things and make better more positive choices in all areas of your life.

You will find the most comprehensive goal-setting exercise at the end of the book. That's when it will be most effective, as you will have all the skills and knowledge you need to make it happen and the goal is really just a strategy of how to get there, a bit like planning a route when you have a clear destination in mind. Before we get to the part where we even start to think about how much weight you need to lose, I would like to clarify my own position on how much weight you 'should' lose. I have a standard answer whatever your shape and size:

You need to lose enough weight to live (and thrive) in a healthy body that enables you to do whatever you want without physical restriction.

Personally I am not a fan of skinny, I don't think it looks healthy and it can be as unhealthy as being fat. Curves are good. Some models look to me like they need a good pie. Whenever I talk about being fat, I am only talking about being fat enough to affect your health and your lifestyle. There is a distinct difference between being curvy and slim, which is desirable, and being skinny, which is definitely not. Females especially – I am talking to you!

The Human Brain

Your brain is changing every day. It is a constant work in progress, think about this statement: you can never step in the same river twice. If we think of the River Thames, we can step in what we call the River Thames every day, but each time we step out and step back in again, different water molecules are touching our legs and some of the river bed will have moved. It will not be exactly the same; although it looks as though it is the same river, it is constantly changing. Your brain is exactly the same. As you read this book you will be making small and significant changes even before you do the exercises, as you will be building a strong awareness that what you have been doing is causing you pain, and you can learn new ways of thinking that bring you pleasure instead. All of this is happening inside your brain through a process of thoughts that create your mind.

The mind has been described as, 'What flows through the brain'. We can't see our mind or our thoughts, but we can see the effect of them.

If you dropped this book then you know it would fall downwards to the floor. This is the predictable effect of gravity; we can't see it, but we know it's there and we can accurately predict its consequences. With the right equipment we could weigh and measure the book and know not just that it would fall to the floor, but calculate how long it would take and with what force it would land. If we dropped it from a greater height, we could measure how that would change the speed and velocity.

Thoughts that create your mind are like gravity in the sense that they have measurable outcomes. If we take food as an example of one of the things you think about every day, then if we know how many times you think about making 'good' versus 'bad' choices, we can predict if your size and shape is going to stay the same, increase or go down.

It's estimated we make around 200 food choices per day, and that ninety percent of these are made by our unconscious minds; thoughts that we have had so often in the past that they have become so automatic we are not aware we are even having them.

The human brain is made up of several components working together as one unit. The individual cells are called neurons. These each have two ends that spread out into tiny strands called axons, or dendrites, and a thin strand connecting them together. A message is received by the dendrites at one end and passed down the cell via the axon to the axon terminals at the other end. The message then gets passed on to the dendrites of the next neuron. In this way information is transferred. This isn't as simple as one small connection per cell, each neuron has approximately 5,000 connections.

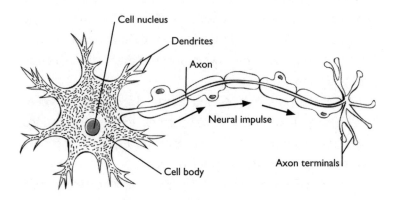

How a neuron works

The signals passing between the neurons have to cross tiny gaps called synapses. Neurotransmitters carry the messages across this gap from the axons of one neuron to the receptor sites on the dendrites of another (just like a ferry takes a car across water). These neurotransmitters (ferries) are either excitatory, which means they activate a response and the message is passed on, creating action, or inhibitory which means the signal is repressed and inaction is the result. When it comes to food for example, they either say 'eat' or 'don't eat'.

Neurons fire 5–50 times per second and each individual signal is a piece of information. That's a phenomenal amount of data, far more than any computer could handle, and it's all under your control.

Looking After Your Brain

In the nutrition section you will learn how what you eat can affect this process, as the neurotransmitters that send messages are made of specific amino acids (proteins) and the receptor sites are made from essential fatty acids (EFAs). Without the right nutrients you cannot build the right structures anywhere in your body, including your brain. What you eat chemically influences how you think and feel.

The human brain has evolved over time and has been likened to a building of one floor that has been extended with additional floors added above. Each area or floor has a specific function in terms of survival and emotional functioning.

Your brain weighs around 1.3kg (3lb) – around two per cent of the average body weight – and accounts for 20–25 per cent of the body's total energy expenditure. The energy the brain uses is glucose. Sadly it does not burn fat for energy at all so, although your thoughts can make you slim, it's not quite in the way you might have hoped!

When we are born our brains are rough drafts or sketches. During infancy we go through a 'critical stage' where our brains are chemically predisposed to learning quickly. This is why we can process so much and why so much of our fundamental belief system is created before the age of six. In recent years, new technology has enabled us to understand more about how our brains function when it comes to behaviours and habits and we have discovered just how plastic and adaptable the brain is. As with the river analogy, it is constantly changing through a process called neuroplasticity.

Your Brain as a Sat Nav

The process of learning involves creating new neurological connections, which are called 'maps'. We have a neurological map for everything we do, for example, we have a neurological map of how to walk, ride a bike, write, play an instrument, drive a car, clean our teeth and literally everything else we do. The more we use these maps, the stronger and more hard-wired they become.

We need these maps because our brains are always looking for the easiest route. When you first learn something, the amount of activity at the synaptic connections is huge, as you process and perfect the most efficient way to achieve the task. Many different axons connect to numerous different dendrites in a particular pattern, creating a unique map. Once you become more accomplished, your brain chunks down the process (just like creating a zip file in your PC to make the file more compact) and uses less connections to achieve the same task, creating more brain space for the next experience. If it did not do this, we would have to relearn everything each time we did it. Imagine if every time you got behind the wheel of a car it felt like the first time you had ever driven, or every time you got on a bike you had to learn how to balance all over again.

Child's Play

Babies have 50 per cent more synapses and, as we grow into adults, a massive pruning occurs because our brains become more efficient and learn to 'save' a wide range of programmes as neurological maps.

During our early years (one–six years old) our brains are at their most plastic and exposure alone is enough to create new neurological maps; in other words, just being in a new situation results in learning, without something having to be formally taught to us. In adulthood however, exposure alone is not enough to illicit neurological change, we must be focused and attentive on the task at hand, or we must associate massive emotion with the experience. It doesn't matter if the emotion is pleasure or pain. We have maps for things we love and things we hate, and are constantly trying to steer a course away from pain towards pleasure. If we want to make wilful change and overwrite an existing map (i.e. habit), a state of high emotion or focused attention must be evoked. When we deliberately and consciously create a new map it's called self-directed neuroplasticity (SDN). This is what you are going to learn how to do. Imagine – you can become your own brain surgeon!

Emotion and repetition are the keys to rewriting old maps and, when these are used, change can be fairly quick. In 2000, Eric Kandel won a Nobel Prize for showing that neurons can double the number of connections with repeated stimulation, and later showed that, if unused, they begin to shrink within three weeks. In simple terms, if you stop doing an old habit, after three weeks you will get neurological change in the form of a weaker map; if you then associate pleasure with an alternative habit, you will create a new stronger map. This is the basis for all the exercises in this programme; you will be remapping your brain.

Self-directed neuroplasticity has the power to remould and change the brain, and once new maps are created they can become rigid. This is because trained neurons are faster and clearer than untrained neurons so they outcompete other maps. This means that the new habits you can create if you genuinely follow the exercises in this book, and absorb the many suggestions in the text both consciously and unconsciously, will be stronger than the old ones, giving new meaning to the phrase, 'Change for good'.

Creating New Maps

Babies use association alone to determine what something means. Although adults also use association to give things meaning, the process is more complex with us as we have additional influences i.e. beliefs, values, emotions, past experiences, judgements and likes/dislikes.

The key area for formative learning (deep in the forebrain) is permanently 'switched on' up until the age of around eleven. From late adolescence onward, it only switches on when one of three conditions occur:

- A novel situation
- A shock
- Intense focus, maintained through repetition or continuous application.

In short, for babies neuroplasticity is effortless. During adolescence we have another period of enhanced plasticity, this is why teenagers are so impressionable; but as adults, we have to work at changing our brain.

Enriched environments stimulate and promote brain function and growth, and more barren environments, by their nature, do not. Your brain is much like a muscle in that you really do 'use it or lose it'. In a muscle the 'use it' component is movement in the form of exercise, in the brain the 'use it' part is electrical stimulation via the thought process. Thoughts are like biceps curls for your brain.

If you want to strengthen your biceps – do a bicep curl. If you want to strengthen a new habit or map, use a positive thought. Remember, just like gravity, a thought is a thing that has a predictable outcome.

The brain has often been compared to a computer, but in reality it is nothing like a PC because it can change and adapt itself. It is more like a living creature with a large appetite. It wants to be fed so it can grow. Your brain doesn't just learn, it is constantly learning the best way to learn.

Brains are by their nature opportunistic, adaptive and resourceful. They are also vulnerable to outside influence, both positive and negative.

Self-directed Neuroplasticity (SDN)

You are constantly being programmed every day of your life so you might as well get involved! SDN helps us to understand how we can do this.

Modern technology has allowed us to map brain activity in response to a range of different stimuli. When patients are wired up to a scanner and shown alternating images of puppies, dirt, kittens, bricks etc. different parts of the brain light up in response to the different images. This teaches us how things make us feel and emotion is a key driver for behaviour, as we will find out.

What we can also see is how much a specific area of the brain is used for a given task, and this can then be measured during and after repetition. One of the early examples of this is was when one of the pioneers of SDN, Dr Pascual-Leone, mapped blind subjects learning Braille. They studied five days per week for one hour 45 minutes, with an hour's homework. Braille readers use their fingers to feel combinations of dots, so they use their motor skills to move their fingers and their sensory cortex to process what they are physically feeling. He found the more they learned, the larger the brain maps for their reading fingers became, and that there was a clear relationship between the size of the finger map and the amount of words learned.

Pascual-Leone also discovered that there is a cycle that involves periods of learning followed by periods of consolidation as, after a few months, there seemed to be little or no apparent improvement in learning. However, the scans showed the newly created maps becoming more refined and established over this time, in other words, becoming stronger.

In another experiment he taught two groups of people who had never studied piano a sequence of notes, showing them which fingers to move and letting them hear the corresponding sounds. They were then divided into two groups:

Group one played the exact same notes for two hours per day for five days.

Group two did not physically move but visualized themselves playing the same five notes, also for two hours per day for five days.

Both groups were mapped daily and at the end of the five days the group who had only mentally rehearsed the notes produced the same physiological changes in their maps as the playing group. This shows the importance of mental rehearsal (visualization) to master a given task. We can apply these same principles to behavioural change. If we combine these processes with what we know about inducing emotional states (i.e. different ways of feeling) and changing brain wave activity (more about this later), we can significantly shorten the period required for change. When it comes to brain function, we cannot tell the difference between an imagined scenario and one that actually happens; imagination is reality, and brings about very real neurological change. The exercises in this programme make use of this important fact.

The first law of plasticity is known as 'Hebb's Law', and states that when neurons repeatedly fire in the exact same pattern to create a map, they become wired together, making that habit or response automatic.

'Neurons that fire together, wire together.'

Stages of Neuroplasticity

1. New neurological pathways or 'maps' are created

2. Maps are refined

3. Fewer neurons are required to complete the initial task (pruning)

4. Speed and efficiency improves

Brain maps are highly competitive. If we stop using a specific map, other maps will quickly move into the space using those same neurons to control other skills. This is called 'competitive neuroplasticity'. To demonstrate this, Pascual-Leone totally blindfolded sighted subjects, excluding all light from entering their eyes. Within two days he found the part of their brains that processes images (visual cortex) changed its 'job description' and began processing tactile and auditory information instead, showing clear plasticity. After five days, when the blindfolds were removed, the previous mapping and activity resumed. This further enforces the 'use it or lose it' principle.

This is useful information because the neurons used for your old eating habits (the ones that made you put on weight!) will redefine their job description and role when you stop the old behaviours, giving you an opportunity to create brand new maps for a whole new set of eating habits. Providing you continue these new thoughts and habits, the old maps will die off through natural pruning, and the new maps will become stronger.

There is an endless war of nerves going on inside our brains. If we stop exercising our mental skills, we do not just forget them; that space is turned over to other skills or movements we do instead. We get more efficient at doing what we do, whether it's good for us or not. This is why world-class athletes and musicians practice the same drills over and over again; they cannot afford to reduce their level of competency, even by a fraction. If you are highly trained at responding in a certain way to cakes, biscuits, chocolate and other heavy, fattening foods, and eat them whenever you see them, it becomes automatic and you will naturally be drawn to this response until you decide to change it. You can't just cross your fingers and hope that one day these foods lose their appeal; you have to actively change your brain. The good news is, it's easier than you think.

Once the 'critical period' of childhood development has finished, our neurological maps are to some extent set. When we learn a 'bad' habit, it creates a brain map and every time we repeat it, it claims more control of that map, preventing that space being used for 'good' habits. This is why, traditionally, unlearning is much harder than learning, and why learning 'the right things' at an early age is so important.

When a guitarist repeatedly uses two fingers to play the same note, the individual finger maps come together, wiring the fingers to work as one unit, controlled by one map. It becomes almost impossible to move just one finger; the neurons are so used to firing together. The good news is that with the techniques in this programme, you can accelerate the process of change, and as you have already learned, the new maps will be stronger than the old ones.

As you will learn later in the book: habits are not broken, they are simply changed. This is because the opposite of Hebb's Law also applies;

'Neurons that fire apart, wire apart.'

When you stop doing something, it feels different and often confusing. This is the pruning effect of neurons dying off; however neurons are competitive and compete to stay active. This can create a craving for the behaviour you are trying to stop because the neurons will be trying to re-establish the failing map. You need a stronger, more positive, counter thought to collapse this craving and associate pleasure with doing the new behaviour instead.

While other body cells need food to grow, neurons need stimulus; this comes in the form of a thought. Thoughts both feed the brain and shape it.

What we call 'memory' is simply a neurological record or map of everything that has happened to us, which is what helps us to make decisions. We can artificially create new memories and maps that 'sprout' new neurological connections.

If you are wondering how long it takes to change, try this exercise.

Exercise
. . . .

Stand up with both arms outstretched in front of you at shoulder level and clasp your hands. Notice which thumb is naturally on top. Now separate your hands and open your arms wide, then bring your hands together again but, this time, put the other thumb on top. Focus and deliberately notice what you are doing and how it feels to clasp your hands this way. Then release and open arms wide and repeat again with your favoured thumb on top. Then repeat again with opposite thumb on top. Keep alternating for 20–30 seconds until it feels less uncomfortable to change thumbs. After 30 seconds it might still feel different but it will be noticeably easier as, even in this short time, you have created a new map. It's important you actually do this exercise, rather than just read it; firstly, because it shows a level of commitment and proves to yourself that you are actually planning to do the exercises, and secondly because we learn by doing. In doing this exercise, you will have a physical learning experience of just how quickly new patterns can be formed, and old established ones become easier to ignore.

. . . .

Before You Start

There are many practical exercises in this book that work best if you use the accompanying journal. You can download a PDF of the journal, plus some additional material, by visiting www.theplacebodiet.co.uk and clicking on the link at the bottom of the home page. If possible, do this now, as you will need it in a few minutes.

Exercise

Before you begin, take some measurements so you can accurately monitor your progress at certain stages of the programme. First, weigh yourself on some reliable scales. These must be the *only* scales you use in the following months, because scales vary according to how they are calibrated and where you position them, and your weight varies depending on what time of day you weigh yourself, so all these things need to be consistent and repeatable.

Next, get a tape measure and measure the areas shown on the table in your journal (shown below). If possible, get someone to do it for you. Record the measurements in the full size table in your journal.

DATE	WEIGHT	ARM 1	ARM 2	BUST	TUMMY	HIPS	THIGH 1	THIGH 2

This is one of several exercises to accompany this book that you can also find in your free journal, available to download from www.theplacebodiet. co.uk via the link at the bottom of the home page. I cannot overstate how important this journal is, as it will be your personal record not just of your progress, but also of how your brain works.

When you measure yourself, make sure the tape is level and not twisted. *Always measure at the widest point for each body site*: there's no point measuring your waist if below it you have a bulging tummy – that's why the table says 'tummy' and not waist! For some people, the widest point for the tummy measurement will be on their belly button; for others (depending on where they store their fat), it may be several centimeters below. It's the same thing with your hips – technically, you would take the measurement in line with the end of the pubic bone, but adapt this if this is not your *widest point*. When you measure individual thighs, do exactly the same thing.

You can't beat noticing that your clothes are getting looser, so, in addition to measuring yourself, find a pair of jeans or trousers and a top that are currently too tight for you and try them on every week so that you can see a real difference. Remember, scales can be unreliable and your body weight can fluctuate by 1.8kg (4lbs) within any given day, so you *must* use other measures of your progress to get a balanced view of your progress.

....

I recommend that you do not repeat any of the measurements, including your weight, until you have completed the (optional) two-week, Healthy Quick-Start Two-Week Plan in Chapter 15. After that, measure and weigh yourself once a week at the most. You don't need to weigh yourself every day – this is not a strict diet in that sense, it is a plan for your mind and body that will get you to a healthy place physically that just happens to include being a healthy weight. How you approach the programme mentally is vital to your success. If possible, get together with a friend, or a small group of friends, at a set time each week to take the measurements. Research has shown that the support of a group can be very beneficial. I must add though, this is only the case if the overall mental attitude is one of support and encouragement. It is not a chance to get together for a right old moan. Be disciplined and use the group only for encouragement and support, and for sharing ideas.

There are a couple of places in the book where I will ask you to think about what you want to achieve but, as I've stated already, the most powerful goal-setting exercise comes at the end. It's at the end for a reason; by the time you reach that point you will have read and done the exercises, and you will understand which foods to eat by using the simple colour-code system. When you have all this information you can create your own personal strategy. Although you will be making changes as you go along that will result in weight loss, the final goal-setting exercise will really bring everything together and make the changes you want to keep, permanent.

. . . .

PART I

How Your Mind Works

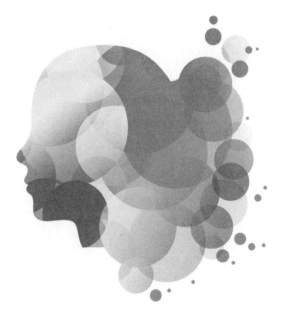

Chapter 2

How Are You Feeling?

Exactly why are you reading this book? Just take a moment to consider that question properly. If your answer is something like, 'Because I am fed up with being fat and I want to be slim', how do you know that's what you want? Seriously, how do you *know?*

Consider this concept – you don't 'have' feelings, you 'do' feelings. Take love, for example. Think of a person, or a pet, or even a thing that you love deeply. Would you say, 'I *have* love for them', or would you say, 'I love them', making love something you *experience* or *do* rather than *have*? Forget the rules of English grammar for a moment, and think of feelings as verbs, in that you *do* them as opposed to *have* them. Now think about how you are 'doing' knowing that you want to be slim. At some level, that 'knowing' is based on a feeling.

The 'why' question when embarking on a new project, especially one that is going to require you to make some changes, is important. If you haven't got a strong enough 'why', your efforts will wax and wane until they fade away completely. You will learn much about the concept of pleasure versus pain in this book, and as humans this is a key part of our motivation strategy. You must always have a clear understanding of why you want to lose weight, what will happen if you do? Versus what will happen if you don't?

The term 'hearts and minds' is very relevant here; you need both working together to make change not only possible, but also enjoyable and rewarding. The 'heart' part of your brain is your limbic system. This is the part of your brain that operates solely on feelings and emotions and is a powerful driver of behaviour, but does not process language; that's the job of your neocortex on the floor above. This is where you work out your 'how'. In a clinical setting, when electrodes are used to stimulate pleasure centres (PCs) in the limbic system, the subjects experience a state of euphoria. PCs are a key factor in the reward system. In animal studies when the PCs are turned on, the animal can learn new tasks more quickly. This may explain why so many of us are best at the subjects we enjoyed the most at school, where the learning was fun, stimulating and taught by our favourite teacher, not just as children, but also in terms of what we remember or find interesting as adults.

In summary, 'why' has to come first; I will help you to find your 'why' and then I will show you 'how'.

This book is going to teach you so many exciting things about how you 'do' feelings. We are taught that we process all the information we receive through our senses in our brains, and of course, technically, that's true. However, there is also a clear mind–body connection that ensures we transmute (change and adapt) those chemical brain processes into sensations and feelings in different parts of our bodies. For example, have you ever felt weak at the knees? You don't have a brain in your knees, so how is it that you can feel something there that is based on an emotion? We know we have nerves in our knees and that they tell the brain when our knees are hurt, that makes perfect sense, but how can an emotion create a feeling in our knees that literally makes them weaken or wobble? There are other emotion-based sensations that present themselves as physical symptoms, including butterflies in the tummy or tension headaches.

Your Mind Affects Your Body

The reality is this: there is on-going, non-stop communication between your mind and your body. You are *one* unit made up of *two* different corresponding parts, and here comes a really important point: one of those parts is much more powerful than the other.

Your *mind* can directly affect the health of your body. Your mind also drives your behaviours and your body is simply a visible representation of what has been going on in your mind – all your thoughts about yourself. Put simply, you (and everyone else) can see the effects of what goes on in your mind by looking at the state and shape of your body. If you constantly think, 'I can't be bothered', you are likely to have a different body shape from someone who thinks, 'I will make the effort'.

In modern medicine, the body has long been treated as a totally separate entity from the mind, often at great cost to the patient. Louise Hay, the founder of Hay House (who publish this book), was one of the very first people to recognize that our thoughts and our feelings affect our health in very specific ways – either positively or negatively – and that we can use our minds to change the health of our bodies. Today, many others are following in her wake, developing new ways of thinking and behaving that can positively impact on our health – physically, mentally and emotionally. Recently, the ground-breaking American scientist

Bruce Lipton wrote *The Biology of Belief*, an astonishing account of how our thoughts *literally* change the biology of our cells. Dr Joe Dispenza overcame serious injury using the power of thought, as explained in his great book, *You Are the Placebo*. The idea that our minds affect our bodies had been dismissed as 'New Age' thinking for years, but it can now be proven at the chemical level, right down to changes in DNA. I will teach you much more about this later in the book.

Turning Information into Action

Let's look at how your emotions drive your behaviour. If you have two opposing feelings, the strongest of these will determine how you behave. It's not possible to feel good and bad at the same time, because one feeling will dominate. For example, you want to be slimmer than you are now, yet a part of your mind still wants the feeling it gets when you eat too much or get comfort from certain heavy fattening foods. Up until now, the latter has been the dominant feeling and that's why you are overweight. Do you want to change that feeling now? Are you ready?

Exercise

Stand in front of a full-length mirror with as few clothes on as possible. Spend a few minutes (or as long as it takes) having a good look at yourself as a physical being. Allow yourself to acknowledge all the things you don't like about being fat. You may think, 'I just hate it!' but try to consider exactly *what* it is that you hate. For example, you might think: 'I hate getting undressed in front of someone', or 'I get out of breath whenever I go upstairs', or, 'I can't buy the clothes I want' or maybe you can't take a child or a grandchild swimming because you don't want to be seen in a swimming costume? You get the kind of thing. Now make a list of the top six things you hate about being fat and write them in the in the following table you will find in your journal (available from www.theplacebodiet.co.uk). Leave the second column blank for the next part of the exercise. Make sure you start each point with, 'I hate'. Things you just 'don't like' won't have the emotional clout to work for this exercise, so be really honest with yourself.

When we look at the power of awareness later in the book you will see why this exercise is so important, but so that you can start getting benefits and making changes right now, I have put this exercise here. As soon as you get one answer keep asking yourself, 'And what else?'

WHAT I HATE ABOUT BEING FAT	HOW THIS MAKES ME FEEL
1. I hate how I look	1. It makes me feel embarrassed and ashamed (then ask yourself – and what else?)
2.	2.
3.	3.
4.	4.
5.	5.
6.	6.

Now think about how each of these things makes you *feel*. For example, 'Getting undressed in front of someone makes me feel ashamed and embarrassed', or 'Getting out of breath makes me feel unhealthy', or 'Not being able to buy the clothes I want makes me feel frumpy'. When you have identified the *feelings* you associate with each of the six things you hate about being fat, write them down in the second column. Make sure you start each one with, 'I feel'. As soon as you have identified one feeling, ask yourself, 'And what else?'

Why do you think that, despite hating these feelings, you have still been *doing* the behaviours that make you fat? The answer is that you have been distorting reality to fit existing ideas and beliefs, and making wrong associations.

The next step is to identify six things that you've been doing on a regular, even daily, basis that have been making you fat, and keeping you fat. Your answers might be: 'I eat chocolate and sweets every day', or 'I keep eating even when I've had enough', or 'I buy and eat junk food', or 'I dish up more than I need', or 'I sit down too much instead of being active – I'm lazy', or 'I eat fast without thinking about what or how much I'm eating'. Spend some time now and honestly identify what your *behaviours* are. Write them down in the table below, making sure you start each one with 'I' so you can begin to take responsibility and associate deeply with what you are learning. Remember, this is all about *you*! Leave the second column blank for the next part of the exercise.

BEHAVIOURS	DESIRED FEELING
1. I eat when I am not hungry	1. To feel comfort and pleasure
2.	2.
3.	3.
4.	4.
5.	5.
6.	6.

Now think about the *feeling* you get when you are 'doing' these behaviours, or more importantly, the feeling you *want* to get! For example, you might say: 'I want to feel comforted', or 'I want to feel full and satisfied', or 'I want to feel as though I don't care about being fat'. Write your answers in the second column. If you can't think of a feeling – think again! All behaviours, big or small, generate a feeling of some kind, and doing nothing is, by default, doing something. Often, especially with comfort eating, the desired feeling is to feel numbness – to blank out the negative thoughts you are currently experiencing. Whatever the feeling is, it ends with 'and happy', otherwise you wouldn't want to feel it. Even if you do something that makes you feel *unhappy*, there's some benefit in your feeling unhappy and that makes it a worthwhile feeling.

· ·

Do You Want to Harm or to Heal?

Have you ever stopped to ask yourself how you actually benefit from this kind of eating behaviour? Would you suddenly get a knife and slash away at your arm to relieve boredom, or to feel comforted? Of course not – that would be madness! There's a name for that type of behaviour – self-harming – and it's a symptom of great mental distress. Well, I have shocking news for you: overeating and making your body fat is a clear case of self-harming! In fact, in some ways, it's even worse than the more obvious forms because it's insidious. That means it's sneaky and deceptive – it's self-harming by stealth. It's so stealthy that you can convince yourself you are not self-harming – but you are. Let me say that again, in another way:

Every time you overeat or drink high-calorie junk, especially when you don't need food for energy (i.e. when you are already satisfied), you are deliberately harming yourself.

Overeating is no better or no different than self-harming with a knife – you just kid yourself that it is. When you harm with a knife there is clear evidence of the harm in the form of scars. But look again, you can hide a scar somewhere on your body with clothes or make up, but you can't hide your whole body completely, even with the baggiest of clothes; so your excess body fat is clearer and more visible than any scar could be. It's a sign to you and everyone else that you are self-harming, possibly every day.

It's time for some honesty now. When you eat to numb emotional pain, or because you don't think you are worth the effort it takes to be healthy, you are using the same technique that an alcoholic or a drug addict uses to bury, numb or forget an unpleasant feeling or difficult circumstances. Rather than changing their circumstances, they artificially and temporarily change how they *feel*. The trouble is, when they regain normal consciousness they crave a return to the escapism of drink or drugs. Instead of dealing with their problems, they amplify and add to them. Being a 'foodaholic' might not sound as bad as being an alcoholic, but believe me when I say it is – if not worse. Shocked? If so, good! It's time for a wake-up call. Remember this:

Overeating is not a form of escapism – it's self-harming.

Some people are 'professional victims' of life's problems, deriving pleasure from feeling unlucky and unhappy because it defines them. Does being fat define you? Is it *who* you are, or is it *what* you are? Think about this question and write your answer down below:

Being fat is ....

If you think it's *who* you are, then you are wrong. Being fat is not who you are, it's merely *what* you are, and you can start to change that right now. Being fat is a physical symptom, or indicator, of your behaviours, in the same way that a scar is the symptom of a past trip or fall. But while some scars are for life, being fat does not have to be for life. It does not define you unless you choose to let it, and opt for becoming a victim. I doubt that this is the case with you, though, because you are reading this book. That tells me (and you) that you want to change and that you want to know how to do it. You are already learning how.

Exercise

Now I want you to think of ways of generating the feelings you want through behaviours that are *not* self-harming and fat-making. This exercise is something you can return to again and again, as certain things can make you happy on one day, but not on another. For example, if the feeling you want is 'to escape', or to 'feel numb' in order to avoid a negative thought, watching a movie or a natural history programme like *Planet Earth* might be the perfect way to take your focus away from you and on to the bigger picture, which is a good thing. However, if it's a gorgeous sunny day, shutting yourself indoors to watch TV may not be the best idea. Similarly, if you want to feel happy and you love walking, taking a hike may have the desired effect in fine weather, but if you make yourself do it when it's cold and wet, you may end up with a different feeling than the one you want!

As you think about this, try to come up with a variety of ways of generating the feelings you desire. I've given some examples below; write your ideas in the blank columns in your journal. We will build on this when we look at the habit loop later on. Each chapter will build on the one before, making the learning and progression as easy and natural as possible. There is a purpose to every single exercise included so, if you complete them in order, over the next few days or weeks you will be able to change limiting beliefs and old habits that you may have had for years.

DESIRED FEELING	ALTERNATIVE BEHAVIOURS
To escape	Have a long soak in the bath with an inspiring book; visit/call a friend
To be in control	Make or create something – write a poem, paint a picture make a healthy meal/snack from a recipe
To be happy	Listen to music; look at photographs of happy occasions; call or visit friends; go for a walk
To spoil myself	Have a pampering beauty treatment; go somewhere special (not food related)

Now, it may seem like I'm pointing out the obvious here, but there's a good reason for this, so bear with me. You need to start believing and accepting that if you want to look and *be* different physically, you have to *do* different things. This becomes easier if you take some time to think about what you can do *instead* of overeating that will still give you the feelings you want.

The problem with the whole concept of dieting is that people do things that they don't enjoy in order to reach a goal. Then, when they get there (assuming they can do what they don't enjoy for long enough), they naturally stop doing the things they didn't enjoy and the weight goes back on. This is because all the reasons they overate in the first place are still there and they haven't come up with an alternative behaviour to meet those needs! But *you* are not going to make that mistake – you are going to address this issue of changing your body by changing your mind – for good. Is that what you want?

Exercise

Before we go any further, let me ask you just what it is that you want to achieve with this programme? I mean specifically, which dress size do you want to be? Or for men, which trouser size? Write your answer below:

CURRENT DRESS SIZE	DESIRED DRESS SIZE

I have deliberately not put weight as a goal here, and I will explain why later on in the book, although we *will* take weight into account. We will also add a time frame to this, but for now, focus clearly on what you want to achieve and start to believe it will happen. Start to see in your mind (or visualize) how you will look and feel a month *after* you have achieved your goal, once you are enjoying all the benefits. Then visualize yourself three months after that, then six months, so it is not the actual achieving of the goal that is first and foremost in your mind, but the months *after* you have already achieved it. As you visualize, make sure you take notice of your new behaviours. What do you see yourself doing now you have made the changes and lost the weight? How is it different from how you behaved before?

• •

There are two especially important times for controlling your thoughts and feelings, when you can most easily influence and change your behaviours. They are: just before you go to sleep, and as soon as you wake up, when you are in an 'Alpha State' and your brain is most open to new suggestions.

Tuning in: Brain-wave Frequencies

The many electrical impulses passing between neurons collectively create an enormous amount of electrical activity. This can be measured using EEG and other scanning equipment, and has enabled scientists to monitor which areas of the brain receive the most blood flow and are therefore the most used during a given task or stimulation. The level of brain activity can be measured in 'brain waves' and each quantified level is associated with a specific state or level of alertness.

GAMMA	27hz and up	'Zen state'; being 'in the zone'; formation of ideas; language and memory processing; learning; peak mental and physical performance.
BETA	12hz–27hz	Awake; processing sensory data and trying to create meaning. People lacking sufficient beta activity, experience mental or emotional disorders, depression and insomnia

ALPHA	8hz–12hz	Awake but relaxed and not processing much information. When you close your eyes and 'go inside' you automatically start producing more alpha waves and your internal world consumes your attention.
		Consolidates information and helps recall memories; lessens discomfort, pain, stress and anxiety; *ideal state for plasticity.*
THETA	3hz–8hz	Light sleep or extreme relaxation; 'twilight' state.
		The veil between conscious and unconscious thins out so there is very little conscious awareness. A very receptive mental state for hypnotherapy.
DELTA	0.2hz–3hz	Deep, dreamless, unconscious sleep.
		A restorative state: the body is healing itself and 'resetting' its internal clocks.

When you are relaxed, your brain uses alpha waves and as a result, you are more creative and better able to use your imagination. You have already learned how vital your imagination is in the process of change through the pianist's imaginary study mentioned earlier (see *pages 15–16*), which teaches us that if you can see yourself doing something in your mind in a powerful way, then you can also do it 'in reality' and create a new neurological map. If you visualize in this way often enough, what you are seeing in your mind actually *becoming* your behaviour; you are changing your mind.

This can go one of two ways as some people do this all the time with negative thoughts and projections. How many times have you heard someone mess up and then say, 'I *knew* that would happen!' They manifested the event through negative visualization – they focused on the worst thing that could happen, literally made a movie out of it in their minds, created a map and then wondered why it happened! The technique of visualization must only be used with *positive* visualizations, and as you do this repetitively and with purpose, watch how you can change your 'luck' from bad to good. If you imagine how hard it will be to stop eating certain foods…. guess what! On the other hand if you imagine making the changes easily then the process will be more automatic and pain free. So as you are dropping off to sleep, see yourself in your mind's eye not just being slim, but also doing the things that made you slim with ease and looking very happy.

From today onward, dedicate the first and the last two minutes of everyday to manifesting your goal and setting your intention. Remember to visualize yourself *after* you have achieved your goal actually doing the things that made you slim. If you know, for example, that you are going to work and you have to walk past the vending machine – mentally rehearse walking past it and happily not choosing the heavy foods such as chocolate or crisps that made you fat. See yourself in complete control and happy, perhaps eating something else instead. If you know you are going out for a meal, visualize the restaurant and what might be on the menu and see yourself making a healthy choice and looking happy. When you come to do it 'for real' you will find it feels much more natural. For athletes mental rehearsal is every bit as important as their physical training, and you are no different.

To help you do this, use the visualization guidelines in the journal (if you haven't yet downloaded it, go to www.theplacebodiet.co.uk and download it now).

Two Minds, Two Brains

There are many things in your body that you have two of, apart from the obvious arms and legs; you have two lungs, two kidneys and two reproductive organs (ovaries and testicles); even your heart is effectively two separate pumps working in unison. As you will learn, you have two minds, a conscious and an unconscious mind, but you also have two hemispheres of your brain. Unlike the two sides of your heart, these two elements are connected, and communicate with each other. Many people are either right or left brain dominant and each has its own characteristics. It's commonly reported that left brainers are analytical and like to process carefully. Right brainers, on the other hand, are more likely to be described as creative and don't need fine detail to make a decision, they can see the bigger picture. In reality, no one is solely one or the other, we are using both all the time.

When it comes to changing your mind, a basic appreciation of the differences between the roles of the two hemispheres is useful. Take a look at the two lists and see which one you most identify with.

Characteristics of the Right Brain (RH):

- Does not process time – it's always 'now'
- Thinks intuitively – no rules or regulations
- Explores possibilities
- Spontaneous, carefree
- Perceives the 'big picture'
- Gives things meaning
- Understands how things relate to each other
- Empathetic
- Understands non-verbal communication; i.e. what is meant, not what is said
- Creates 'new' solutions

Characteristics of the Left Brain (LH):

- Puts info from RH into timely succession, i.e. has awareness of time, past, present and future
- Sequential: organizes and compares information with past experiences
- Linear: can predict what will happen when… .i.e. X *will* make me feel Y.
- Defines and categorizes
- Recognizes patterns
- Deductive reasoning/logic
- Thrives on detail, detail and more detail
- Chunks down 'big picture' into bites of data
- Hierarchical; tells you what your favourite food/colour/car is
- Judgemental: categorizes things as 'good' or 'bad'
- Our internal voice originates in the language centres in our LH, i.e. 'I must do this because…'
- Home of your ego centre, providing you with an internal awareness of you
- Manifests a sense of (internal) authority
- Strives for independence
- Understands verbal language/semantics; processes exactly what is said in a literal sense, i.e. if someone took it 'the wrong way' that's their fault
- Is dominant; when angry it excludes RH brain in decision-making.

The exercises in this programme are designed to meet the design and the needs of both hemispheres. Visualization in particular is a powerful brain changer as you will see, and this takes place in the right hemisphere, especially when we are visualizing a future event.

In the visualization exercises I will emphasize the need to see yourself as if you have already achieved the goal, and are already doing the things that made you slim. This is to put it in past time, so that your left brain, which likes to operate on things that it has already known and are 'proven', neurologically accepts these behaviours as already tried and tested, and creates the new maps. If you only ever see what you want to happen in the future as if it is the future, your left brain is not involved. As your left brain is where much of your strategies are mapped this 'past timing' is vital. In combination with this you must also elicit a powerful emotional feeling of happiness, pride, success, confidence etc. with the image so that it is also recorded in your limbic system. In this way all areas of your brain are working together to create a new mind. If you miss one element out, the exercises will not be as successful. If you are going to do this – play full out and get all your brain involved. Understanding what is happening in your brain as you do the exercises will create awareness and appreciation that what you are doing is working. If, like me, you like to know how and why things work, this understanding will be important to you! If it's not important, do the exercises 'full out' anyway and you will also get the changes you want and deserve.

Harry Potter: *'Is this all real or is it
just happening in my head?'*

Dumbledore: *'Of course it's happening in your
head, but why should that mean it's not real?'*

Chapter 3
Thoughts Are 'Things'

You are a spiritual being. I'm not talking about religion – your beliefs on that are not relevant to this concept. What I mean is that the air around you – the atmosphere or the 'ether' – is not just empty space, it is full of 'information'. And your thoughts are also information – they are real 'things'. Although you can't see them, they have a substance that gives them an energetic force. This concept has become much more widely known in recent years, as films and books like *The Secret* have encouraged people to use their unconscious minds to focus on drawing to them what they desire. This principle is popular, but in reality, in order to draw something to you, you also have to practically do whatever it takes to make that happen. You will learn how to do just that in this book. You will learn how to combine your mental attitude and focus to drive your unconscious mind to create the behaviours that will bring you what you want – a slimmer, healthier body.

This kind of thinking is not new, though. In fact, it first appeared in the brilliant works of the American author Napoleon Hill, who wrote, among other things, the hugely successful book, *Napoleon Hill's Keys to Success: The 17 Principles of Personal Achievement*. Napoleon Hill's works have influenced most, if not all, of today's self-help gurus and the origins of Neuro-Linguistic Programming, or NLP, can be found in much of his work, in particular the concept of 'modelling', which we will explore later in the book.

The First Ever Self-help Guru

In 1908, Hill, then a young journalist, interviewed the powerful industrialist Andrew Carnegie for an article he was writing. Originally from Scotland, Carnegie had emigrated with his family to America at the age of 13. He worked in a factory and in other lowly positions before going on to found a steel company that was valued at $480 million when he retired in 1901. He was the Bill Gates of his day. He then started to give his fortune away to good causes (as Bill Gates is also doing). His strongly held belief was that the rich are merely 'trustees' of their wealth and are under a moral obligation to distribute it in ways that promote the welfare and happiness of the common man. He also believed that anyone could achieve the enormous success that he, and others like him, had enjoyed.

During the interview Carnegie took a liking to the young Hill, and commissioned him to undertake the task of analyzing, and then sharing, the methods he had used so effectively in his business. Hill then spent the next 20 years interviewing some of the most successful people in the USA at the time – including Thomas Edison, F.W. Woolworth and Henry Ford – drawing out and then 'modelling' their thought processes. The sum total of that study appears in his books. I've listed the most relevant principles for you below, because they can be adapted, and are fully relevant to achieving any goal.

Desire – You must create an overwhelming desire to achieve your specific goal. E.g. Associate huge emotional and physical benefits with being slim.

Faith – You must have absolute faith in your ability to achieve your goal. You must believe that you can change.

Autosuggestion – You must learn to accept your own positive suggestion by managing your ongoing internal communication.

Specialized knowledge – You must do whatever it takes to learn any method or technique you need in order to achieve your goal. This book will give you the perfect strategy.

Imagination – Through the power of your imagination, you can create real scenarios and create change. Self-directed neuroplasticity occurs when you imagine yourself doing something new.

Organized planning – You must have a specific strategy. The colour-code system and goal setting exercises at the end of the book will ensure this.

Decision – You must make a definite decision and defeat the act of procrastination. This is also a key part of internal communication and understanding how the brain works.

Persistence – You must develop the ability to continue towards your goal whatever distractions, or temporary lack of success, occur along the way. This is the power of will. Repetition and emotion are the key ingredients in SDN.

The Master Mind principle – This is the driving force of combined thoughts for a common goal. Spend time with like-minded people who are already slim and healthy so that you can mirror their behaviours.

Transmutation – To change one form of energy into another (just like when your voice is turned into vibrations that pass down a telephone wire and are then transformed back into vocal sounds). E.g. Understanding thoughts are things.

Subconscious – The connecting link between our senses and our recording process. E.g. The collaboration of our two minds working together to create new habits.

The Brain – A broadcasting and receiving station for thoughts. You are never not thinking or communicating with yourself. Be careful what you say – you are listening!

Sixth Sense – The means through which 'Infinite Intelligence' (more about this later) can communicate and respond to any individual effort. This entails being aware of new ways of thinking and doing by listening to your body and non-verbal communication; being more observant and instinctive in doing the things that take you towards your goal.

Thinking Outside the Box – If you do what you have already done, you will get what you have already got. Thinking differently and changing your perspective is essential.

We will explore these principles in more detail as we go on. You will learn how to adapt and apply many of them to you, and your desired goal of weight loss. These are well-established, tried-and-tested techniques that have been used by some of the most successful people in the world to help them achieve their goals – most of which were considerably harder than learning how to eat a bit less and move a bit more!

One of the key findings of Napoleon Hill's research was the 'power of thought'. We have already begun to look at this concept on many levels and we will build on this further as we go along.

Your thoughts truly are 'things' and just because you can't see them, it doesn't mean they are not there. Remember – if you drop something, you know the power of gravity will cause it to fall to the floor. You don't question it. You can't see the gravity, but you can see the effect it has. Now you know that your thoughts are just the same – you can't see them, but you can see their *effects*.

Where Your Thoughts and Behaviours Come From

In your conscious mind, you can process approximately seven pieces of information at any one time (plus or minus two). Every other thought you have is in your unconscious mind. Now just think about that for a moment, because a thought can also be described as a 'message' or a 'signal', and your body is a mass of signals constantly passing between your cells and your brain.

Right now, there are trillions of messages whizzing around your body at a very high rate of vibration. They are telling your body when to breathe and how much CO_2 to expel; they are monitoring your blood pressure, monitoring how much blood goes through your kidneys, which cells need repairing or renewing… you get the idea? If you were aware of all these messages, you'd be completely overwhelmed with information, so there is an ingenious, and essential, division between your conscious mind and your unconscious mind.

The illustration below explains, very simply, how the conscious and unconscious minds work. It shows an iceberg: a huge, mountain-like structure with its top *above* the water line and the bulk of it, the bit that determines its strength, *below* the water line. The conscious mind is shown as the top of the iceberg, the tiny bit above the water line; and your unconscious mind – the really important bit – is the major part below the water line.

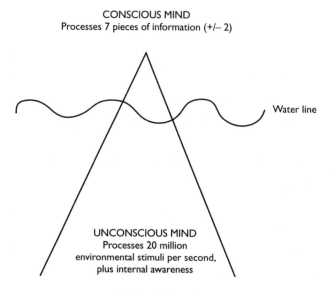

CONSCIOUS MIND
Processes 7 pieces of information (+/– 2)

Water line

UNCONSCIOUS MIND
Processes 20 million
environmental stimuli per second,
plus internal awareness

Your Two Minds

In the previous chapter we looked at 'how' you think and feel. This is done by your 'conscious mind' – the bit above the water line, where you process your environment. For example, as you read this, how comfortable are you? What are your surroundings like? As you focus on the words you are reading now, are you saying them out loud in your head? Are you adding your own comments to specific points? All of these things are in your conscious mind. Below the water line, in your unconscious mind, is a database of everything that has ever happened to you. Some of this information will never reach your conscious mind, but it can still have a huge impact on your thoughts, and therefore on your behaviours. It could be experiences from childhood that you have long forgotten *consciously*, but these have formed your belief system into what it is today, determining how you think and behave.

The 'water line' acts as a filter system that determines exactly what information makes it through to your unconscious mind. When you have an experience, you instantly decide whether the information is worth keeping, and so file it in your unconscious mind, or delete it — millions of minor signals and messages are filtered out in this way. Other experiences, or pieces of information, do get through the filtration process, but only because we adapt or distort them to make them 'fit' a particular belief system.

Creating Associations

By manipulating information in this way, we can sometimes record information incorrectly. A good example of this is when smokers convince themselves that smoking will not cause terrible suffering and disease, and a painful death, even though they 'know' consciously that it will. They delete crucial evidence and then distort what's left, creating different associations to make it acceptable. For example, when young people start smoking they tell themselves, 'It makes me look cool in front of my mates'. This creates a positive association with smoking and the unconscious mind accepts this distortion as true and installs the behaviour. As they get older and wiser, those people learn this is not true consciously, but the unconscious pattern has been set and, until that association is broken, the unconscious belief and the behaviour of smoking persist, despite conscious protests.

All it took to install the negative behaviour (which then became a neurological map) was a *powerful thought combined with a strong emotion*. A thought *without* emotion cannot be converted into a belief or a behaviour — you must have the emotional intensity of *feeling* to connect with the thought — to give it the power to create the behaviour in the physical form of a neurological map. In the same way, to delete a behaviour, you must combine an *opposing* thought with a powerful emotion to delete the connection. For example, have you ever eaten something that made you so ill that you still couldn't touch it, months or even years later? Last year I got food poisoning from a lamb tagine, and every time I see it on a menu now I shudder, and wouldn't consider ordering it. It's all about association.

Here's a simple way of looking at it:

**Thought + intense emotion
= association = behaviours created**

or equally

**Thought + intense emotion
= association = behaviours destroyed**

Below is another 'iceberg' illustration. This one explains how the conscious mind feeds the unconscious mind information in the form of conscious 'thoughts' – passing them through the 'water line' based on the intensity of the emotion, and the associations we subsequently attach to it.

The conscious mind (via the senses and general processing of information) 'sends' information deep into the unconscious mind to be cross-referenced (not unlike an internal 'Google search'), matched and filed in the correct place – i.e. in line with our established beliefs and values. The unconscious mind then collates all this information and, based on what has been received, 'sends' its instructions back to the conscious mind to create and drive everyday behaviours.

You can think of the conscious mind as representing workers reporting into head office (the unconscious mind), which creates policies based on how that information compares with its existing database and then sends back strong signals for how to behave. An important fact to consider is that although they are separate, they strive to complement each other. They will each compensate if it thinks the other is not getting it right. For example, if eating certain foods brings much pleasure and your conscious mind suddenly denies you this pleasure by stopping these foods and replacing them with other foods or things that bring pleasure, your unconscious mind will self-sabotage your efforts. There will always be compensatory actions between the two to maintain balance and strive for harmony. The aim of this programme is to meet the needs, and honour the intentions, of both your conscious and unconscious mind.

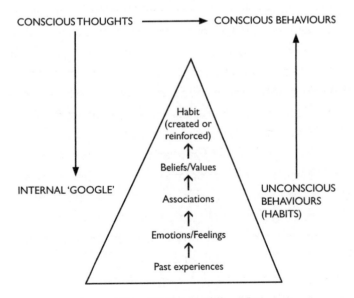

Where Our Behaviours Come From

We can create behaviours using our conscious mind. For example, however you are sitting or lying right now, choose one body part, perhaps an arm or a leg, and move it three times.

If you did it, you will have shown yourself that you can make a conscious decision to move. (If not, try and remember that these exercises are all here for a reason.) That's a simple example of a conscious thought generating behaviour. In your everyday life you are constantly searching for other times that you have been in the same situation and checking-in to see if you already have an automated response (map), in order to save brain power. This is called 'fast thinking' and is a process we often use for food choices.

How Your Thinking Drives Your Behaviour

Later in the book, you'll find an exercise that will enable you to make use of this process to great effect, but in the meantime, here's a way of looking at it in very simple terms. When you were young, your mother told you not to touch the oven because it's hot. Either you believed her, or you actually touched the oven yourself and learnt that if you touch this thing it hurts. Either way, information was combined with emotion and association to create a behaviour – in this case, the behaviour was to keep away from the oven!

This is how you learn everything you now know – by association. Put another way, if you decide something is important then it influences you; if it's not important, it doesn't. That's why when someone you know, or even worse, love, insults you, it hurts more than if the insult came from someone you have a low opinion of, or don't know. What creates the all-important association? You know the answer of course – it's a thought.

When you are thinking about whether or not to associate pleasure or pain with something, your mind processes the associations it has already made. For instance, if someone says to you, 'Let's go to London for the weekend', and your internal Google search engine tells you that you have been to London before, your mind will use that as a reference. If you had a good time on the previous occasion then you will respond positively, and if you had a bad time, you will respond negatively. If you have never been to London, your mind will search for similar experiences and will project what you think will happen over the weekend to make its decision. Simply put: your mind likes patterns – it likes things that are the same. If a particular situation has evoked a particular thought, emotion or behaviour in the past, your mind is likely to stick to that pattern, unless you change your thinking and make new associations. Every behaviour has its own unique map.

This is why so many people stay in abusive relationships – although they hate their situation, they are afraid of being alone, or worried about where they will go if they leave. If they stay with what they know, at least they know what they are dealing with. Have you heard the saying, 'better the devil you know'? Well, that belief is responsible for a lot of people not changing, or not trying something new. We like to stay within our comfort zones; our unconscious mind likes and desires a sense of security and it gets that from doing what it knows. Until you change that thinking, and start to think that things will be better another way, you will be stuck in the rut.

How Much S.H.I.T. Do You Have in Your Life?

It has been said that of the thousands of thoughts we have every day, over 80 per cent are the same negative ones repeated over and over again. So, it's time for some new thinking! You are just one thought away from changing everything. Are you ready for that? Every thought is a piece of the jigsaw puzzle that makes up who you are.

I have been working with people who want to change how they think and feel (as well as how they look) for more than 20 years, and it's my belief that many of the negative thoughts those people had weren't even their own – by that I mean that they accepted the negative imprint from someone else. In other words, they accepted other people's thinking as their own. My advice to you is to stop letting other people's Systemic Harmful Invasive Thoughts (S.H.I.T.) affect you!

Systemic – goes all the way through you

Harmful – hurts

Invasive and **I**nfectious – gets below the skin

Thoughts – are *Things* and they define you

These types of thoughts activate the amygdala and pain centres in the brain, altering your brain chemistry and making you feel bad.

It's their S.H.I.T. not yours; you can create a much better thought process of your own. So the next time you find yourself thinking something negative, just remember: that thought is S.H.I.T.; choose a better one. Your internal voice is a representation of your thoughts and as such, it can be controlled and changed. Most people leave their internal voice on the default setting. They play what they are used to hearing – what they know. They don't make the effort to tune into a different voice; you would probably retune a radio and see what else is on if you didn't like what you were listening to, so do the same in your head.

If you really *must* accept other people's thoughts, then surround yourself with positive, optimistic people who really achieve what they want. I'm not talking about money, although that often comes to positive thinkers, but in all areas. Physically, who has what you would like to have? Listen to what they say. Talk to them in a bit more detail about how they think. Pay attention to their actions and notice how many more positive choices they make around food. Are they just lucky to be slim? Of course not; there's no such thing. It's all down to choice.

C.L.E.A.N. Thinking

Here's an alternative way of thinking. Use language that is:

Caring

Loving

Encouraging

Aspirational

Nurturing

These CLEAN thoughts increase serotonin levels and activate the pleasure and reward centres in your brain, thereby changing your brain chemistry to make you feel good. When your brain is full of 'happy' chemicals you are predisposed to learning and creating new neurological pathways. We will revisit this when we look in more detail at internal dialogue later on.

You Become What You Think You Will Become

Your thoughts define you. You must have had the thought, 'I want to be slimmer', or you wouldn't be reading this book, but you *are* reading it. I invite you to continue to read... but do it patiently. Stop and pause regularly to reflect on what you are learning. This is not a novel, although it does tell the story of *how you became you*, and what you can become if you really want to. Of course, like all good stories, it leaves you to fill in the really important bits! So, as you read patiently – and possibly more slowly than you would normally read a book, allow your thoughts to form – you might just awaken a genuine interest within your mind about how to change. As you take the simple steps and complete the exercises, know also that *how you think as you read will determine your success with this programme*. If you think about it, this could be the very last time you ever have to consciously make the effort to get the body you want. That could be both an incentive and a relief, depending on how you think about it!

Can you remember how exciting learning something new was when you were young? To a child, even learning to walk is exciting. As children, we don't process the thought, 'I keep falling over – I'll never be able to walk, I'm a failure!' We just keep getting up and trying again until we learn from our experience, adjusting our balance until we can not only walk, but run, dance, hop, skip and jump, too! It's no coincidence that when you were a child you learnt at a much faster rate than you do now. As we mentioned, the subject you most liked at school was probably taught by your favourite teacher; he or she made learning fun and interesting, and inspired you.

Recreate that teacher, or a new persona that is equally as inspiring, now, as you read through the pages of this book, and let the knowledge and understanding unfold. With every page you turn, open a new page in your mind with pleasure and anticipation; be eager to learn and as eager to please yourself as you might once have been eager to please your favourite teacher! 50 per cent of everything you need to know about how to change and be the person you want to be, physically and emotionally, is in this book, the other 50 per cent is already within you, perhaps hidden or buried. As you read, your own 50 per cent will be revealed to you through your thoughts. It might come to you piece by piece, or perhaps in one big epiphany moment! I wonder which way you think it will happen? I hope that by now you are curious about exactly how you will change, as (far from killing the cat!), curiosity results in exploring and creating new mind maps.

Exercise

Think about the negative thoughts you've had on a regular basis that allowed you to self-harm by overeating and under-exercising. Are they your own S.H.I.T. thoughts? Or are they someone else's S.H.I.T. thoughts? Who made you think, and therefore feel, that you weren't worth the effort it takes to have a wonderful, healthy, vibrant body? A friend? A relative? A partner? A teacher? A parent? The media? If the influence didn't come from someone else (and it probably did, even if you don't realize it yet) then what S.H.I.T. thoughts did you generate *yourself* that allowed you to abuse and overwrite your instinctive desire for survival and health?

In your journal (download from www.theplacebodiet.co.uk) complete the table shown below, write the name of the person who gave you the S.H.I.T. thought, what the thought was, and what has been the outcome of keeping that S.H.I.T. thought.

PERSON	THOUGHT	OUTCOME
Fred	I am not good enough	Eat for comfort = fat
Me	I am stupid	Might as well be fat and stupid = overeat

The original thought was accepted with such emotion (even if it was a negative emotion) that it became a belief that generated its own set of behaviours. You are just one thought away from changing that – or have you already started to think differently? We will look at beliefs in a little more detail later on, for now, focus on changing your thinking and your associations.

....

How 'I Can't' Becomes 'I Can'

I told you earlier that your mind likes doing things that are familiar. Well, now I'm going to guide you through the process of change. Before you decided that you wanted to change, were you going along thinking there wasn't really a problem with your weight and size? There's a stage before the change process and it's called 'Unconscious Incompetence'. This means you are really bad at doing something (in this case looking after your body) but you don't yet realize it or, more likely, you don't yet admit it. Have you ever worked with someone who is hopeless at their job but who thinks they are great at it? That's Unconscious Incompetence. (You only have to watch TV talent shows to see more examples of Unconscious Incompetence.) While you are at this stage, no changes can take place.

Then comes a lightbulb moment – perhaps you see an unflattering photograph of yourself and you suddenly realize you are bad at something (in this case looking after yourself), but you don't know how to do things differently. This is a moment of acute awareness called 'Conscious Incompetence' – you are bad at looking after your body, but now at least you know you are bad at it and you can admit it. This is a good stage to be at because it can be a springboard for change, as long as you want to change. In fact, without awareness of a need to change – change cannot happen. At this point you need some intervention, some help or information that will tell you how and what to change. You are reading that help right now! When you learn new techniques, like the ones in this book, they don't become automatic right away. In fact, your unconscious mind might even resist change and try to draw you back to what you know. (As explained earlier, this is when fading neurological maps try and fight to preserve their existence by creating a craving or an urge for that behaviour.) If your unconscious thinks you are going to go on a diet, and it has negative associations with past attempts, this may be quite a strong pull back to old behaviours. That's why it's so important to create new associations.

This means that, at first, you must consciously make the changes – you must literally think about doing the new behaviours in place of the old ones. This stage is called 'Conscious Competence', which means you can do it, but only when you think about it. This stage feels different; some people say it's hard, but it's not hard; climbing Everest is hard. Another word I hear is it feels 'uncomfortable'; walking on sharp stones is uncomfortable. The Conscious Competence stage is not uncomfortable either, but it is different. It feels different at first, but very soon (within a few weeks or less) you get used to the new behaviours. Right at the beginning of the book I asked you to do the exercise with arms outstretched, hands clasped, and then to open you're arms and clasp the hands the opposite way. If you did this (if not do it now, or do it again now anyway) then you will have noticed that something that feels different can feel a lot more natural even after 30 seconds of repetition. In the same way, all new behaviours eventually become automatic with repetition. When you reach this stage, you will automatically use the new behaviours instead of the old ones, without thinking consciously

– this is called 'Unconscious Competence'. You have now rewired your thinking and changed your default setting.

Here are the stages again:

1. **Unconscious Incompetence** = unaware of behaviours

2. **Conscious Incompetence** = aware of behaviours

$$\downarrow$$

New Skill, Information and Exercises (e.g., this book's contents)

3. **Conscious Competence** = think to activate the new behaviours

$$\downarrow$$

4. **Unconscious Competence** = automatically do the new behaviours

A good example of this process takes place when we are learning to drive. At first, we have to consciously think about *everything*, the clutch, the gear shift, the accelerator, the visual checks – it's almost overwhelming! But think how quickly after you passed your test you began to drive at the same time as chatting or listening to the radio. You went from consciously generating the thoughts you wanted to doing them automatically, without conscious thinking. Riding a bike is the same: most of us learnt with the help of an adult or stabilizers helping us to balance, but once we had experienced how to do it, and created a physical map for which muscles to move, and how to balance and pedal at the same time, we could do it with ease. Even if you haven't ridden a bike for many years, once you get back on, a few minutes of wobbling is all it takes to reactivate the neurological map and remind you.

Doing It Without Thinking

What other things are you so good at that you can do them without thinking? How many times do you go and get something heavy and fattening to eat 'without thinking'? That's Unconscious Incompetence. The new thoughts and behaviours you are generating right now in your conscious thinking will become automatic the more you exercise them. If you only had one driving lesson per month, how long would it have taken you to get to Unconscious Competence, compared to if you'd had two or more lessons per week? In the same way, the more effort you can put in right now to changing the thoughts you are having consciously, the quicker you will automatically, and seemingly without effort, start making the choices that will give you the body you want.

Through this process – and being aware that you can choose to change – you truly have free will. This means you can stop being the victim of your programming, especially as it's probably other people's S.H.I.T..

It's not about willpower, it's about wilful thinking, but you get to choose your thoughts, so stop listening to the same old S.H.I.T. and start thinking consciously. Think of this as a course in learning to drive – but one in which you learn to drive your brain rather than a car. Your only limitation is what you think you can achieve. As Henry Ford once said: 'Whether a man thinks he can or thinks he can't, he is probably right.'

Just knowing something isn't enough to actually do it, though. After all, you already have a pretty good idea of what to eat, or what not to eat to lose weight, don't you? Of course you do. Later in the book, I will introduce you to a really simple way of thinking about foods that will help you to put into practice everything you've learnt. No more 'eating without thinking'. Remember this:

> *'Knowledge is knowing a tomato is a fruit;*
> *Wisdom is not putting it in a fruit salad.'*

Did you ever look at a tomato and think, 'That would be lovely in a fruit salad!'? Probably not, which shows that the thoughts you apply to what you learn determine your behaviour.

• •

Chapter 4

The Chemistry of a Thought – Become an Alchemist

So, now you know that you are only ever a thought away from getting what you want. You know that a thought is a 'thing', and that it has an energy and a force – just like gravity – even though you can't see it. Now for the really cool bit – when you project your thoughts out into the 'ether' (the word for the universal space around us) as powerful visualizations, images and words, then you can begin to make changes you never dreamt were possible. You will find opportunities opening up for you as you begin to attract a more positive influence into your life.

Your Thoughts Are Energetic Signals

When the Italian inventor, Guglielmo Marconi, told his friends he had discovered a way to transmit sounds through the ether without wires, they had him arrested and taken to a mental asylum for examination! Yet, in 1909, Marconi shared the Nobel Prize in Physics with Karl Ferdinand Braun 'in recognition of their contributions to the development of wireless telegraphy'. Radio waves were initially called 'etheric' waves, because they pass through the ether. Thought waves are not dissimilar to radio waves and, as with radio waves, our thoughts contain information that has been up-scaled; information that can be communicated at a level beyond human speech or vision.

Wherever you are, have a look around right now. What do you see? Furniture, people, trees? But what's in the space in between those things; in the space you can't see? Have you ever thought of this space – or 'ether' – as a conductor of information? Sounds a little crazy? Think again. When did you last make a call on a mobile phone? How do you think the sound of your voice reached the person you were talking to? Did you see the words leave your phone and fly through the air? Of course not – but they did!

How does this happen? Well, everything in life vibrates (or resonates) at a certain frequency, and the ether responds to these varying levels of vibration and exchanges information. In a phone call, it exchanges the information of the sound of your voice between the phones. This is possible because in the 1870s the Scottish scientist Alexander Graham Bell, the inventor of the telephone and an expert on vibration, believed that it was possible to send messages or 'information' through the ether. Today, thanks to his work and his understanding of 'vibrational energy', when you make a phone call the sound of your voice is 'scaled down', or transformed into a vibration that can be sent through the ether, picked up by a receiving station, and 'up-scaled' to become audible words and sounds once more. Pretty cool, huh?

If your thoughts are signals that are transported through the ether, then, I have two questions for you:

• What thoughts are you putting out there?
• What thoughts are you receiving back?

The quality of the thoughts you transmit will determine the quality of the thoughts and experiences you get back through a process Napoleon Hill called 'Infinite Intelligence'. This is your own unconscious connecting with an invisible force that combines and communicates with the etheric intelligence of all the messages and information 'out there' in the universe. In other words, it's the theory that everything you need to know is available to you via something you can 'tune into'. This is commonly known as the 'sixth sense'.

Positive vs Negative Thinking

Have you ever noticed how some people seem to attract bad luck? You can bet that almost *every* thought they have is negative in nature – blaming something or someone, or feeling sorry for themselves. They are stuck on the same frequency and the more negativity they put out, the more of the same they get back. They often suffer physically too, as their bodies take on the negativity to generate illness or disease.

On the other hand, positive people are seen as having better luck: they attract good things and opportunities just seem to land in their laps. Born with the same potential as anyone else, a positive thinker can go from the humblest of beginnings (as in the case of Andrew Carnegie) and by a process of positive thought – combined with desire, persistence, planning and actions – achieve anything they want. Did Andrew Carnegie have any bad luck along the way? Of course he did! He made mistakes just like anyone else does, but he learnt from them and moved on – quickly. He looked for solutions, he learnt to think laterally, and most importantly, differently. Eventually, he found a process that created a lifelong philosophy for him and, through

Napoleon Hill, he shared it with anyone who cares to read it – and everyone should.

If you could meet someone who knew Carnegie or Hill, you would not hear them described as 'a moaner' or as a person who was 'always complaining'. That kind of S.H.I.T. thinking was not in their philosophy. Instead, they developed a strong communication with their unconscious minds through the power of autosuggestion and self-hypnotic language. These techniques enabled them to develop a clear and definite purpose for what they wanted to achieve, and then to devise a strategy to achieve it.

Say What You Want – Because You Are Listening

Self-hypnotic language and autosuggestion are highly effective ways of communicating with yourself. Let me explain a little about how they work. We can think of our brain waves as a bit like tuning a radio or transmitter: depending on the frequency, we can send or receive different signals or information that can't be transmitted on any other frequency or level. For example, when you tune your TV into the History Channel, you can't expect to get MTV, and vice versa. By choosing to put ourselves on the right frequency or in the 'right state', we can receive or transmit precisely what we choose.

We know from earlier in the book that our brain waves vary at different times in our growth and development, and in different physical states. This can be measured clearly on an EEG, which records the electrical activity of the brain. When we undergo hypnotherapy for example, the therapist aims to induce a 'trance state' by reducing our brain waves to a lower vibration or frequency, because this is where we are at our most suggestible and receptive.

As we have already seen, our brains are operating almost constantly at this lower frequency from birth to the age of six, then less so to the age of 12 and even less often when we reach adulthood. This explains why children can pick up new skills so quickly while adults often find it more difficult to learn new things.

If you received *negative* messages from your parents or peers at this critical time in your life – i.e. when you were in your most receptive 'state' – you were more likely to accept them as valid and incorporate them into your thinking and belief system, where they dictated your future behaviours. Conversely, if you received *positive* messages, or constant praise and encouragement, during this formative time, it is likely that you developed a totally different, and more positive outlook, self-esteem and belief system. Your childhood environment, whatever it was like, had a profound effect on how you think and feel today.

When I think of this, I'm always reminded of Jodie Foster who, in an Oscar acceptance speech, thanked her parents for all the encouragement they'd given her as a child. She said they had made her feel as if 'every painting I ever did was a Picasso'. How different might her career have been if they'd told her to 'stop showing off', or said that she wasn't very good at anything? The comments and encouragement Foster received as a child had a positive impact in her formative years and have stayed with her for life; luckily for her they were positive messages. Not all of us have had that experience, but as adults we can access a trance-like state and use autosuggestion and self-hypnosis to delete negativity and give ourselves the positive, affirming and inspiring messages we really want to hear.

Even if you had negative messages in your childhood, remember this: it is never too late to reject a negative suggestion. The moment you begin to think and believe it is not true, is the moment you negate its effects completely. If you no longer validate it, then it's no longer true. This is very important, so I'm going to repeat it again and after reading it, I invite you to close your eyes for a moment and take this learning deep into your heart and soul with as much emotion as you can generate.

It is never too late to reject a negative suggestion.
The moment you begin to think and believe it is not
true, is the moment you negate its effects completely.
If you no longer validate it, then it's no longer true.

What Are Your Thoughts Tuned In to?

Any thought accepted with emotion while you are in a trance-like state (whatever your age) will create associations that literally hardwire you to behave or respond to stimuli in a certain way *every time* you are in that situation. Have you ever responded angrily to someone and then said, 'He/she really knows how to push my buttons'? Have you ever looked at a cake, a piece of chocolate, a lump of cheese, or any food and generated a 'need' and a strong desire for it, even though you're not hungry? That's another button you created by combining a thought with an emotion – you created a synaptic pathway in your brain to repeat that message or thought every time you are exposed to the same stimulus. But it only takes an opposing thought, combined with a powerful emotion, to delete that connection and wire a new one.

A nerve is an excellent conductor of electrical current and so is the brain. When the brain's cells send messages to each other, they produce tiny electrical signals in the same way that a radio wave is a disturbance within a quiet or still space. If a thought is a disturbance in the electrical current, then we have a scientific explanation for the power of thought that can be measured (as in an EEG). However, it is the actions or behaviours that result from specific thoughts that give them their real power.

The Incredible Power of Thought

Let's revisit the concept of the placebo effect and how we can use it to change our minds. In his book, *The Biology of Belief*, Bruce Lipton talks about the power of the placebo and gives the example of a study in which patients needing minor knee surgery were taken into hospital.

All the patients were put under anesthetic, but the operation was only carried out on half of them; for the other half, the surgeons made a small incision where the needle would have gone, so it would look like they'd had surgery, but nothing further was done. None of the patients were aware of the study, but the results showed that there was no difference in the recovery rates between the two groups. In other words, those who had the 'fake' operation got better at exactly the same rate as those who had the procedure. The only explanation for this is that they thought they had been 'fixed', and that thought was powerful enough to generate within them a genuine physiological healing process. That thought literally changed the chemistry within their cells to allow them to repair and renew their knees.

In the many years that I've been helping people deal with how they think and feel about themselves, food or a traumatic event, I've found that for this approach to be effective, you must attach *a definite and strong emotion to the thought* – one that is powerful enough to generate change, either emotionally or physically, at a cellular level. If the patients in the hospital study hadn't truly believed the knee surgery would be successful, it wouldn't have been.

The placebo effect is very interesting and brings up another, much less talked about phenomenon – the nocebo effect. This is when people take on board a *negative* suggestion in such a powerful way that it creates illness and disease. If you consider that positive thinking can heal a knee as effectively as surgery, imagine the implications of being told you have something that cannot be cured; perhaps being told that 'depression runs in the family', and that 'it can't be cured – you have to live with it'.

In *The Biology of Belief*, Bruce Lipton tells the story of a physician who gave his patient the diagnosis of a cancer that was 100 per cent fatal. It was no surprise to the physician when, a few weeks after diagnosis, the patient died, as predicted. However, a postmortem revealed a misdiagnosis – the patient's body showed very little evidence of cancer and certainly not enough to prove fatal. The belief that he had a terminal illness generated such powerful thoughts in the patient that he changed his physiology and killed his own body. You don't have to take my word for this. If you want to know more, the references for this and many other examples can be found in *The Biology of Belief* by Bruce Lipton and also *The Placebo Effect* by Dr Joe Dispenza, who healed himself through the power of focused thoughts and meditation after a serious accident that threatened to leave him paralyzed.

'The Miracle Man'

If you want to see an amazing example of the power of positive thought, then check out Morris Goodman, otherwise known as 'The Miracle Man'. Early in 2011, I was privileged to attend an event where he was a guest speaker. In 1981, Morris, then aged 35, was flying his plane when it crashed. He sustained terrible injuries, breaking two bones in his neck – C1 and C2. People rarely survive a breakage of *one* of these bones, let alone both. He survived the journey to hospital, where he and his family were given a bleak prognosis. Morris, however, had other ideas. Although he couldn't communicate at all, he could hear what was going on and he made the decision to recover. He also decided he would regain use of his body and be able to walk again.

Morris began a process of visualization and thinking that would eventually heal him. After some time, the hospital staff realized he was fully aware of everything that was being said and all that was going on, so they taught him to communicate using a system that utilizes blinking to represent the letters of the alphabet. The first thing he dictated was: 'I will walk out of here'. As the months passed, many doctors told Morris that his goal was impossible and that he shouldn't have these thoughts because he would only be disappointed. Morris rejected this negativity and chose to have different, positive thoughts.

One key milestone Morris wanted to meet was the ability to breathe without the aid of a respirator. He was told categorically that the nerves to the muscles that expand the ribs had been severed, and that for him, breathing unaided was a physiological impossibility. Morris rejected this thought, though, and although he didn't know how his body could breathe naturally again, he decided it would. Every night, when the nurses left him to sleep, he started to work with the respirator. Instead of being passive and letting it do all the work, he tried to assist it. At first, he managed for less than a second, but he continued, night after night, to put his mind to creating a way of breathing by using autosuggestion — i.e. by telling himself with absolute belief that he could achieve it. He spent hours in a trance-like state, repeating that suggestion over and over again. After many weeks, he believed he could take a breath unaided and asked the staff to let him try. They told him it was not possible, but he was insistent, and so in the end they agreed, just to pacify him.

Against All the Odds

When they removed the respirator, Morris breathed unaided for over a minute. Everyone except Morris was stunned. The doctors kept saying, 'But it's not possible!' and as soon as he could breathe for long enough unaided, they whisked him off to a laboratory to find out what was going on inside his body. Their investigations showed that he had trained his stomach muscles to do the work of his diaphragm. After more training through the process of thought and autosuggestion, the respirator was removed altogether. It was a similar story with Morris's ability to swallow. Having been tube-fed, he believed he could teach himself to swallow, and he went about it in the same way until, of course, he could eat unaided.

Morris worked his way through all his body systems and his limbs, until, incredibly, less than a year after the accident, he walked out of the hospital. When he came on stage in 2011, it was the first time he'd given a talk for two years because sadly his wife had died. I can't imagine that anyone at the time of the accident thought Morris would outlive his wife – the family were told he wouldn't even last the night. That's the incredible power of thought.

Morris is the most moving speaker I have ever had the pleasure to listen to, and being in the audience was a humbling experience.

As Morris stood on the stage telling us his story – a living, breathing example of the power of positive thinking – it was a painful reminder that the opposite is also true. Please visit www.themiracleman.org and view clips of Morris speaking. If you are following the Placebo Diet at Home programme then you will see this video in one of the lessons. Since his recovery, he has dedicated his life to sharing and teaching the power of positive thinking. Usually, I think 'positive thinking' is a much-overused phrase, and one that most people don't register the power of when they are saying it, but when you watch this man speak, you truly see its power. If you, or anyone else you know, has ever been given a bleak physical diagnosis, then this is a good place to visit to show the doctors what the power of thought can really do. Doctors are in the medical profession because they want to heal, so they will be delighted if you defy unfavourable odds and get well!

Your Brain as a Wi-fi System

So, you know now that your thoughts are incredibly powerful things. You have been walking around with this loaded gun full of negative rubber bullets – probably firing at yourself more than anyone else. If you thought you were firing blanks, now you know that's not the case: *every thought counts.* These seemingly harmless thoughts are creating negative maps and behaviours that are running your life.

Thoughts truly are 'things'. They go outwards into the 'ether' as vibrational energy, and they go inwards to dictate your physiology: your physical, mental, spiritual and emotional health and wellbeing. When you put a thought 'out there' into the ether, where does that information go? As we have heard, Napoleon Hill describes this space as 'Infinite Intelligence'. It's not a religious term – it's simply an acceptance that the universe is, in and of itself, 'infinitely intelligent'. Whether you believe the universe was created by God, or a force or an energy of such immense intelligence that it can manifest anything, including the planet, or whether you believe the universe was created by the Big Bang, the fact remains that the space in which we live – of which we occupy very little – has its own intelligence. There's even space within every cell in your body, so this 'ether' is also within you. It's like having your very own internal Wi-fi system!

When you make a call on your mobile phone, do you hear the words of all the other calls that are happening simultaneously around you? Of course not. Our senses are incredibly limited – dogs can pick up a level of vibrational sound that is beyond us; birds can see minute objects from distances we cannot – but just because we can't hear or see something, it doesn't mean it's not happening. As humans, we are limited in what we can see and hear, and many of us are limited in *what and how we think*, too. It's time to realize that you are the creator of your own limitations. Whatever you truly believe that you *can* achieve (with passion and a strong desire), you can achieve. Stop and take a moment now to think about how you feel after reading the first few chapters. Have you begun to realize that the process of change begins with a thought? What exactly do you believe you can achieve in terms of changing your body from fat to healthy? Write it down now and look at it. Is it what you want to, and believe you can, achieve or have you imposed limitations on yourself?

I truly believe I can achieve ....

....

So, here's what to do with what you have learnt already (and later in the book we will look at how you can use your imagination to do this even better).

You can direct your thoughts in two ways:

- Put 'out there' what you want to achieve; see it daily in your mind's eye.

- Develop an internal thought process that will direct your unconscious mind to a set of behaviours that will give you whatever you want, whatever the obstacles you have met in the past or meet along the way.

Remember, *every thought* has the potential to change the direction of your life. Have you ever seen the movie *Sliding Doors*? In it, Gwyneth Paltrow runs two parallel lives, each totally different as a result of one moment in time when she had a different thought. In one life she catches the train, in the other she doesn't. If you have seen it you'll know exactly what I mean. Her character is on the staircase going down to the London Underground when she hears a train approach and decides to run for it instead of taking her time and waiting for the next one. In one life she makes it, and in the other scenario a young girl steps in front of her, and in that split second she misses the train. Either way, it was the initial thought – 'run for the train' – that ultimately made the difference. Had she walked for the train, the second option would have been the only one. There are *always* choices, and there are always *consequences* to those choices.

Exercise

In order to promote awareness of what made you fat and the new choices that will make you slim, complete the following table in your journal using the example below. Everything that you do that increases awareness, even if it seems obvious, will begin to sprout new neurological connections in your brain.

THINGS THAT MADE ME FAT	THINGS THAT WILL MAKE ME SLIM
Too many takeaways	Planning meals to have after work
Snacking from vending machines	Taking healthier snacks to work
Watching too much mindless TV	Going to the gym 2–3 times per week
Drinking too much alcohol	Limiting alcohol to weekends, and moderating amount
Not stopping when I have had enough to eat	Having smaller-sized portions

Chapter 5

Every Little Thought Helps

A common mistake that people make when they want to achieve a particular goal is opting for the quickest way of getting there. Sometimes quick is good – if you're a sprinter for example, then the fastest possible time is important! But if you want to achieve something meaningful and lasting, quickest is rarely best. This lesson is captured in a classic children's tale that we're all familiar with: The Three Little Pigs.

Once upon a time, there were three little pigs. The time came for them to leave home and seek their fortunes. Before they left, their mother told them, 'Whatever you do, do it the best that you can because that's the way to get along in the world.'

The three little pigs listened to their mother's advice and off they went. The first little pig, keen to get settled straight away, decided to build his house out of straw. He built it quickly and was pleased with himself, but the big bad wolf came by and when the little pig wouldn't let him in, he huffed and he puffed and he blew the house down; and then he ate up the little pig.

The second little pig built his house out of twigs, but the big bad wolf came along, and when the little pig wouldn't let him in, he huffed and he puffed and he blew the house down. Then he ate the second little pig.

The third little pig built his house out of bricks; he took his time and his house was strong. When the wolf came to the house, he wouldn't let him in. The wolf huffed and he puffed, and he huffed and he puffed again, but the house would not blow down. The wolf thought himself clever so he climbed onto the roof to get in via the chimney. But the third little pig was smart – he built a fire in the grate and placed a large pan of boiling water on it. The big bad wolf fell into the boiling water and was no more. The third little pig was safe.

The moral of the story is, of course, that the quick-fix option, although attractive, rarely yields long-term results. Sure, the first two pigs had a house, but not for very long and, in the end, their efforts killed them. Extreme dieting can do that, too.

Lazy Thinking

We have already learned we have two minds, a conscious and an unconscious mind. In addition to that we have two ways of thinking: fast thinking and slow thinking. In his excellent book, *Thinking, Fast and Slow*, Daniel Kahneman describes these two separate processes as individual characters called System 1 and System 2, influencing us sometimes independently and at other times working together. Previous learned associations and conditioned responses determine much of this process.

As you would expect, fast thinking (System 1) is quick and immediate. It does not hang around to calculate the best option in any given situation; it works on instinct and impulse, making instant judgements. It is influenced by emotions and associations, and cannot follow rules. When you see a cake, pastry or whatever heavy food has made you fat, it immediately responds by saying to your slower-thinking mind, 'I've got this one' – and makes the decision for you. If the slow-thinking mind got involved and thought through the consequences, you might not eat it.

Slow thinking (System 2) is more rational, makes deliberate choices and can follow rules. However, it is economical or even lazy; if it can save brain energy by following an established pathway, it will. This means when you ask it a question, it will quite often answer a different but similar question without you realizing the adjustment. In many ways it looks to justify previous decisions by repeating them and adjusting facts to fit a certain belief.

System 1 can never be turned off. If I present you with an image of a cat, then you look at the cat and cannot not recognize it. If System 2 is busy on a task and you are presented with a choice, System 1 automatically takes the responsibility to makes an immediate instinctive decision, without having to bother System 2.

Studies have shown that when subjects are engaged in a cognitive task, such as memorizing a set of numbers, and are simultaneously offered the choice of two desserts, a virtuous fruit salad or a chocolate dessert, they are more likely to choose the chocolate dessert 'without thinking' than they would have been if they had not been engaged with a task. There may be a physical component to this as sustained brain activity requires a significant amount of glucose and the opportunity to replenish stores with sugary desserts would be an obvious choice. The higher the cognitive load (thought process) the harder it is to exert self-control, as self-control is itself a thought process that requires energy. When you are brain fatigued you are far more likely to make poor food choices, largely because your brain has a sweet tooth. However, high blood glucose levels put you in fat-storing mode so that's not desirable either; it's all a question of balance. If you work in a stressful job in which you have to spend many hours concentrating, then this may be relevant (and we will discuss this in the colour-code system later in the book), as low blood glucose makes it harder to stay motivated.

When System 1 believes that something is true, the conclusion comes first and the supporting arguments follow. As a famous American politician once said, 'Never let the truth get in the way of a good story!' System 2 wants to be economical with its use of energy so it will accept the conclusions presented by System 1 to save the effort of checking, rather like a lazy employee taking someone else's word for something without checking for himself. Many commercial mistakes have been made as a result of this attitude, and many people have got fat using the same process.

For weight loss, you need to use more of System 2, in other words slow your thinking. Do not be misled by the word slow, we are talking an extra second or two, not an hour or even five minutes. Just a few seconds spent thinking can take inches off your waistline. Practically, this means that the moment you notice your hand moving towards some food almost without instruction, you should pause, think, and check your choice fits with your values and what you want to achieve.

It All Adds Up

Let's say you are out for lunch with a friend who is about the same shape and size as you. He or she chooses a tuna Niçoise salad and you choose a four-cheese pizza. Does that make you fatter than your friend straight away? Of course it doesn't! You think it's just one little choice that won't make you fat, and of course that *one* choice doesn't. Over the next few months, you meet regularly with this and other friends, and having eaten a greasy pizza and not got fat, the message is, 'One more won't hurt', so you continue to choose creamy coffees, pizzas and high-fat desserts, because hey, *individually* none of these choices matters, right? Wrong! After a few months, an accumulation of bad thinking and split-second fast choices really *do* matter. It's like compound interest!

Question: *How did you get fat?*
Answer: *One bite at a time!*

To sum this section up remember this acronym. It's called T-CUP thinking and is another way of describing slow thinking:

Think
Correctly
Under
Pressure

Any chefs among you will know that to cook a lobster you simply stun it and drop it into boiling water. To cook a frog, however, you need to be subtler. If you dropped a frog into boiling water, it would immediately jump out. However, if you put a frog into tepid water it is quite happy. Then, when you increase the water temperature by one degree it barely notices and can sit or swim quite happily. Increase another degree and the frog is thinking, 'One more won't hurt' and so it goes on, until in the end you have boiled frog. He kept thinking that one more wouldn't hurt, but combined together they *all* hurt, a lot. Don't be a frog.

Every thought matters. You didn't get fat eating one pizza, one chocolate bar, one ice cream or one extra slab of cheese. You didn't get fat not going to the gym for one day or not moving any more than you had to for 24 hours. Your fatness is the result of the compound effect of all your thoughts and behaviours.

Doing the 'Write' Thing

While I was running my health clubs, I completed a Master's degree in nutrition and exercise science because I was convinced the more I knew the more I could help people. For my dissertation I wanted to look at the effects of food recording – of having to write down what you ate – and if (and by how much) this affected food choices. On the basis that to eat it, you had to write it down, I was pretty sure I would find it *did* make a difference. As students we had to follow and experience several different types of diet and as part of that process, we also had to record everything we ate for a set period of time and analyze the results. I certainly changed what I ate, purely because I didn't want to admit to my professor that I had eaten certain 'unhealthy' things. How hypocritical would that make me, as a student of nutrition and sports science? Of course I wanted to be seen as virtuous!

So, I designed my own study to run over 10 weeks and got a group of willing volunteers from within the health clubs, all of whom wanted to lose weight. I told them I'd be analyzing their diets, but I couldn't manage to do them all at the same time, so I asked half the group to record what they ate for the first five weeks, and the other group for the second five weeks. The volunteers didn't know the reason for the study, or what I was looking to prove.

As it was for a clinical study, it was important to remove as many variables as possible, so I asked all my volunteers to attend a nutrition course for an hour a week for six weeks prior to the 10-week programme. I asked them *not* to change what they ate over this six weeks, but to simply use it as a learning experience for the programme.

At the end of the 10 weeks, I analyzed my data and found, as expected, that irrespective of whether they were in group one or group two, the period when they *recorded* what they ate was when they *lost* the most weight. This was all good! But, in addition to that, I was amazed to find that when I looked at the measurements I'd taken when the volunteers signed up – i.e. before the nutrition course – they'd lost more weight over this six-week period than the whole of the following 10 weeks, when they were supposed to be making a more concerted effort to change their diets!

This was in spite of the fact that I'd specifically asked them not to change what they ate during the nutrition course and them all having agreed! When I talked to the volunteers after the study was completely finished and I had my results, they all said they didn't think they had made any significant changes to their diet over the six weeks. It was clear to me that they had made small, possibly even unconscious, changes here and there, based on what they were learning about food and how the body burns fat. These small, non-deliberate changes resulted in significant weight loss for almost all the volunteers. These changes were little things that were so easy to do that they did them every single day and didn't even notice they were doing them.

The good news is that although the changes can be small, when they are repeated often enough they become hugely significant. I will teach you everything I taught my volunteers, and more, later in the book, and you can be even more successful than they were. I have also massively simplified the process of food recording, as you will see with the food record cards. All you have to do is tick a box in one of four colour-coded columns; it takes just a few seconds yet the effects on learning can be profound.

Increasing Your Awareness

Why did my subjects make changes they didn't even know they were making – and then deny all knowledge of them? The answer is – awareness.

I mentioned earlier that you will make some changes just by reading the book, in addition to the more significant ones you can make as a result of the practical exercises. This is because your unconscious mind becomes aware of certain things, and begins to change some of its previously held beliefs and associations accordingly. A few years ago very few people ate kale, it was just another leafy green vegetable; now, however, it is one of the most fashionable foods going and hundreds of thousands of people have brought juicers or blenders and are making kale-based smoothies. Not because it's a nice colour – in fact the colour of the smoothie resembles pond water! It's because of the awareness of the associated health benefits. It's an easy and cheap way to get valuable nutrients into the body.

There are many foods that you currently associate with pleasure that are, in fact, causing you massive pain. Similarly, there are plenty of delicious foods that could genuinely bring you pleasure but you are associating them with dieting, which itself has negative associations for many people, maybe you included. Anything that you associate with pain, you will eventually stop doing. This is why I asked you to complete the table in the previous chapter.

There are many triggers that elicit fast-thinking, impulsive or automatic food choices. These can be anything, such as places, words, images or people. In psychology, the term used for something that triggers a response is a 'primer'. If a trigger elicits the likelihood of a known outcome that is pleasurable, then the chances of you repeating that behaviour is very high. A thought is capable of bringing about a reflexive response, outside of your awareness.

The purpose of most advertising campaigns is to prime you to reach for a particular product in a specific situation. But everyday life contains many primers that you may not even notice. In 2014, McVitie's spent £12 million (according to their press release) researching what we associate biscuits with, in order to produce a brand-new advertising campaign for existing products such as Digestives and Jaffa Cakes, already two of their bestsellers. Their marketing director said, 'Biscuits are utterly trivial, yet they are immensely powerful. Imagine a world without biscuits. It would be such a cold, sad place'. To illustrate this point they created some cute, cuddly images to ensure we associate comfort with these foods.

In one of the adverts the cuddly animal in question was a kitten, but there were other more subliminal associations that were intended to act as primers or triggers. If you are following the online programme along with the book then you will see the advert in one of the videos but, if not, imagine this scene:

The advert shows a group of happy (slim) nurses, seemingly on a break from work in a hospital setting. The lucky ladies are laughing and 'ooooing and aahhhing' as they open a packet of digestives and out comes a kitten: cute. The strapline is: 'The chocolatey snuggle of McVitie's', and the last shot shows the ladies enjoying a bite of their biscuits. The actual biscuit is on screen for barely a few seconds.

Just take a moment to think about the implied associations in the advert:

- Kittens – comfort
- Hospital – health
- Nurses – health
- Smiling group – friendship
- Smiling group – happiness
- All slim – health
- Background music from *Fawlty Towers*, a cult comedy TV show – fun and laughter

This is how easy it is to be primed or programmed by someone else. If you are eating digestive biscuits because you think you will feel comforted – then you have been had by the marketing company. No doubt, when they look at their bank balance, they are feeling a lot more comforted than you are after eating the biscuit.

The reasons these adverts work is because they have a lasting effect. Long after you have seen the advert, if you see a packet of McVitie's you unconsciously remember the kitten feeling, and you get a physical desire to feel comforted. The same goes for numerous situations in your life, and not just those that are food related.

In one study, posters intended to prime a specific response were placed above a tea and coffee station in a workplace where there was an honesty box for contributions so that staff could then make their own refreshments. The first poster was a pair of eyes, implying, 'I'm watching you' and the second poster, the following week, was a bunch of flowers. In week one, when the poster with the eyes was displayed, the average contribution for a drink was 70 pence. In week two, when the flower poster was displayed, it went down to 15 pence.

You can use this information in a practical way to encourage slow thinking and increase your instinctive awareness: print off the picture of the eyes in your workbook, or any other eye images you have, and place them on the cupboards where you have the heaviest fat-storing foods: maybe on the cake or biscuit tin, or perhaps on the cheese box in the fridge. Even though you will know you are being primed, it will give you the momentary reminder that you need to consider making another choice. It's an amazingly powerful exercise. Just do it.

....

Chapter 6

'Brain Juice'

By now the message is clear – you have to change your thinking. A negative thought works in a stealth-like way; it goes unnoticed because of its small size, but it quietly combines with other S.H.I.T. thoughts to bring about a bad situation, physically or emotionally, or both.

Let's go back to the inspirational Morris Goodman. Do you reckon he thought sometimes, 'I won't practise my breathing tonight – one night won't make a difference'? Absolutely not! That S.H.I.T. thought would not have been allowed to enter his mind. He thought about how to breathe unaided *every* night, until he *could* breathe unaided by a respirator. He had a clear and definite purpose and a plan to achieve it. He thought about how to swallow *every day* and visualized himself doing it until he *could* swallow. He thought and visualized his limbs into action *every day*, until he resumed full use of them. He achieved all of this despite his doctors telling him that what he dreamt of was not physically possible. In Napoleon Hill's success principles he was personifying the acts of desire, faith, autosuggestion, decision, persistence and transmutation, and utilizing his subconscious mind in a very powerful way. Luckily, you only have to put in a fraction of this effort to heal your body from fatness and save your life.

Unsuccessful people (just like the frog) think that small, individual decisions do not matter. Successful people (just like you are now) understand the compound effect of positive thinking. If you change all the little things you eat, and stop making the bad choices that make you fat, then you will be slim. It's not rocket science, is it? But it *is* a process: you must focus on how much you are *changing your mind* before you focus on how much, or how quickly, your body is changing. I promise you with all my heart, when you replace the way you think about food and activity with a more positive collection of thoughts and actions, your body will soon begin to show you the compound effects of those changes. You won't become a frog.

The changes are easy to make because they are usually very small things. But the problem is – it's also easy, if not easier (because it's what you know), *not* to change. You have to choose – that's free will. Other than your genetic skeletal structure, *you* get to choose the size and shape of your body. So which shape do you choose: fat and heavy, or slim and healthy? Think carefully because there are consequences to either option.

The 'Brain-juice' Diet

Your brain uses different chemicals to generate different moods or feelings. Let's call this chemical cocktail 'brain juice'. By training your mind, you can literally change your 'brain juice' to change how you think and feel and, as a result, behave. To illustrate the point, let's look at how our 'brain juice' affects hunger and what actually causes some people to compulsively overeat. Always keep in mind that hunger is a primitive survival instinct that makes us seek food. Remember also that we still have the same genetic make-up that we had when we were hunter-gatherers and had to forage for food. Our chemistry and physiology have not yet adapted to the fact there's a supermarket on almost every corner and food is available 24/7. The process of generating an action to seek food occurs within your brain's chemistry (or 'brain juice'): it is altered in response to internal signals from your body, and from external stimuli in your environment.

Your hunter-gatherer ancestors didn't sit on a rock watching hefalumps go by and say, 'Ooh, I fancy one of those, with large fries!' They hunted what was available, *when* it was available. Overeating didn't exist. Theirs was a hugely physical lifestyle, so inactivity was not an option either. You won't find cave paintings depicting your fat ancestors: obesity didn't exist.

If you consciously restrict your food intake to the point of starvation, your survival instinct will eventually kick in and, just as you cannot ignore the need for sleep, eventually you *will* eat. This is what happens, to a lesser extent, when you follow a strict, low-calorie regime; it's like surviving on two–three hours of sleep instead of the required seven or eight – you can do it for a while, but there's a tipping point at which your body demands sleep. If you semi-starve yourself with strict calorie restrictions, then at some point your unconscious mind will take over and drive you to eat. This drive is so strong it often causes bingeing, and the feeling of gratification is then so great that extreme pleasure is associated with bingeing.

You have already learnt, and will read again repeatedly, how important associations are when it comes to creating behaviours. Remember the illustration of the iceberg (see page 49)? Have a look at it again now as it clearly shows how experiences, when combined with strong emotions = behaviours. One extremely emotional event can be all it takes to create an association powerful enough to generate a behaviour that can be triggered over and over again, any time you are in the same situation.

Many overeaters think about food almost all the time; they are constantly on full alert for supplies! This is an exaggerated survival response. It's a bit like a phobia, which is a normal, rational fear that has been amplified out of all logical proportions. Your conscious mind tells you *logically* that the spider/cat/dog won't hurt you, but in your imagination you create an alternative reality that triggers a specific physiological fight-or-flight response – a change in your 'brain juice'. A compulsive eater has the same exaggerated process in response to the need for food. When people constantly or regularly overeat, they think about food and what they could/should/would like to eat, pretty much all the time – except when they are eating. Ironically, when eating, they often just shovel the food in, sometimes even deleting the tastes and textures in their rush to get the satisfaction of having eaten it, and that brings temporary relief. This is an important point so I'll say it again:

> *It's not a specific food you crave; it's the feeling that food gives you. You are craving a feeling – not a food.*

This happens through a mixture of the basic primal need for food, and the internal associations and anchors you associate with the food.

The 'Brain-juice' Cocktail

Of course, there are many chemicals that make up our 'brain juice', but this is not intended to be a biology book, so I won't go into all of them. It's helpful, though, to look at the two most significant chemicals that are associated with cravings (whether it be for food, drugs or even gambling), because it will become clear to you why you have certain feelings and responses. These chemicals are dopamine and serotonin. We need both in different situations, and they work in opposition to each other, countering each other's actions to achieve balance.

Dopamine – This chemical is involved in numerous bodily functions, including balancing hormones, blood flow and the intestinal process of digestion. It is a survival hormone that increases alertness, and our ability to focus and process information. In an emergency, it can even be converted into adrenaline. It's important for motivation and striving to achieve a reward.

Serotonin – This works in the opposite way: it decreases our alertness and aids relaxation. When serotonin levels fall too low we can become irritable and can easily be overwhelmed by every day stressors. High dopamine and low serotonin creates the perfect environment for cravings and other compulsive behaviours. A rapid intake of carbohydrates can temporarily raise serotonin levels bringing a tangible physical relief, but in the long term, this inhibits regular serotonin production. So, despite the quick-fix highs, carbohydrate binges have long-term negative consequences. The more carbs we eat, the less seratonin we produce naturally, which means we are driven to eat more carbs to make more – and so begins a very vicious, harmful and fattening cycle. Good-quality proteins contain tryptophan – a large amino acid that converts to serotonin in the brain, stimulating natural and balanced serotonin levels. A diet too high in protein, however, can also inhibit serotonin production. It's all about balance. (More about how to achieve this later; I have done all the working out for you and put it into the colour-code system you'll find in Chapter 14.)

Why Do We Overeat?

Hunger and the drive to eat are naturally occurring processes. In fact, they're lifesaving, so why does eating, or more specifically overeating, become an issue with some people and not others? It's all down to 'brain juice' and the process of learned associations. When a slim person looks at a fat person and watches them eat when they are not hungry, they can't understand it. They say things like, 'If she really wanted to be slim, she would just eat less.' But it's not quite as easy as that – not without some mind-aerobics and some good techniques.

Think of a newborn baby. Its brain receives an internal signal that food/energy levels are running out and need to be replenished. The baby gets a signal that it can't consciously process as words, but it gets a feeling that means, 'I want food'. This creates an unpleasant physical sensation, or pain, that causes the baby to cry. Mum hears this cry and her breasts, full of milk, swell in response to its cry. She feeds baby and both are satisfied and relieved of the pain – and at the same time, a strong emotional bond is formed. Food brings a relief from pain. That is one of the key drivers of all behaviour – the avoidance of pain. Baby learns that when it sees or smells mum, food is at hand, and it anchors that comforting sensation with food and its mum. Even if you were bottle-fed, the process is the same – apart from the breasts! You are in pain, you get a hunger signal, you eat – pain relieved, positive associations made. The cycle is complete until the next time fuel and energy levels are low – it's a continual process.

Under normal circumstances, this cycle works well. But if you are a compulsive eater, a mixture of bad 'brain juice' and associating pleasure with heavy unhealthy, fatty, sweet or generally high-calorie foods, means that the drive to eat is activated even when you are not hungry. Pain (not just physical pain but emotional pain, too) can also be a motivator to eat: studies have shown that when rats have their tails pinched and experience pain, they continue to eat, even though they have been fully fed. Not unlike some humans I know who eat in response to pain. Do you?

Eating when you're not truly hungry in response to other factors (emotional, environmental or physical) is like any other reward-driven, addictive behaviour. It is no different to the gambler or the drug addict getting his 'fix' from his chosen poison. It's learned behaviour, driven by 'brain juice'. In a recent article, Dr Steven Novella (an academic clinical neurologist at Yale University School of Medicine) discussed the historical ineffectiveness of 'dieting', saying that 'Research conducted over the past decade has demonstrated that the sensory experience of palatable food can easily override homeostatic controls of energy balance, leading to overeating in the absence of true physiological hunger.' This is a very academic way of saying that our thoughts can override our natural hunger/satiety signals.

Do You Think Before You Eat, or Eat Before You Think?

For the first time, we are beginning to see a clinical approach to the understanding of what drives behaviour, and that obesity is a symptom of irrational behaviour that can be chemically driven via 'brain juice', and not a cause in itself. I am hugely grateful for this kind of research. For years, I have been working with people to help them change how they think about what, when and how much they eat and I have always believed the solutions lie in the head and not in the mouth! I have had to deal with all the fads, gimmicks and promises made by so many diets – high this, low that, etc. But I now have the technical material to answer many previously unexplained questions about why people overeat, so I can give you a complete guide to changing how you *think* in order to change your body.

Thoughts change your chemistry – emotionally and physically. They can literally change the cell environment so that it heals and repairs – or so that it fails and dies. *You* get to choose – that's what *free will* is all about.

I don't like the word 'willpower'. People talk about it as if it's a 'thing'. You must have heard someone say something like, 'Over Christmas, I just lost my willpower and gained three kilos!' Well, I have news for you – *willpower is not a thing*. It's not like your car keys, which you put down somewhere and then can't remember where you put them. We have *free will*, which means we have the ability to choose our thoughts and behaviours. That is never, ever lost. I've heard many failed dieters blame their lack of success on their lack of willpower – as if it was nothing to do with them! That's a cop-out based on denial and deletion of fact. Whether you succeed or not is entirely down to the choices *you* make – you can't blame anyone or anything else. *You* and you alone are responsible no matter who you live with, where you work or live. It's your body and it's your sole responsibility to look after it. Try not to prioritize someone else's wants or preferences over your right to be healthy.

Get Juicing

To generate new 'brain juice', you must generate new thoughts. You must become a thought chemist. Just as a chemist blends different substances together to create a beautiful new perfume, you must now begin to experiment with new thoughts – and blends of ideas and beliefs – that will give you *a definite sense of purpose*, and a genuine faith in the fact that you will achieve your physical goals. Not can – *will!*

Faith is an essential ingredient in the process of permanent change. I am not talking about a religious faith; I am talking about faith as being a level of knowing, much deeper than belief. Dictionary definitions of faith include: 'Confident belief in the truth, value or trustworthiness of a person, idea or thing' and 'Belief that does not rest on logical proof or material evidence.'

When I think of faith, I'm reminded of a scene in one of the Indiana Jones movies where our hero has to reach a cup containing the magic potion necessary to save his father. He can see it across a great divide between the rocks and he has a 'clue' that requires him to 'Step out in faith and the path will appear'. He takes this literally and, as he steps out in complete faith across the chasm, a bridge appears beneath his feet and takes him across the divide. This is the kind of faith *you* must develop in your own ability to achieve your goal. You must step out and allow the bridge to appear – you might be surprised by how brave you are! Your new bridge will be made of thoughts that are supported by strong, positive associations.

To develop faith you must first create a clear and definite image of you having achieved your goal. You must manifest this image every day until you can see it clearly in your mind. Please don't tell me you can't do this! You might not be able to at the first attempt – Morris Goodman didn't take his first unaided breath at the first attempt either, but he kept going until he got what he wanted! Every time you find yourself saying, 'I can't', you need to tell yourself to 'shut the hell up!' 'I can't' is a pathetic phrase when you think about it: now you really know the power of thought, use what you have learnt to get what you want. After all, that's why you're reading this book, isn't it?

Exercise

Create a strong image of yourself as slim and healthy, and as already having achieved your goal. Generate this image first thing in the morning, as soon as you wake up. Make this 'you' the first person you say hello to everyday. Visualize 'you' throughout the day. See a successful 'you' popping up here and there regularly, and saying hello. As mentioned previously when we were learning about the significance of brain waves, you must also focus on this image last thing at night, before you go to sleep. *Do not underestimate* the power of this manifestation of your successful image – it's one of the most important steps in the process of change, if not *the* most important.

It is important when visualizing that you see 'you' when you have already changed and are reaping the benefits. In this way you store future information in your past. This makes future choices more recognizable because you've seen them before. Things that are recognizable are easier to notice. Have you ever brought a particular make or colour of car, and then suddenly begun to see them everywhere? This isn't because suddenly everyone had the same idea as you, but simply that the cars are easier to notice because you have brought them into your conscious awareness.

Modelling

Modelling is an NLP term (Neuro-Linguistic Programming) for imitating the actions of someone who has already achieved what you want to achieve. It works well in therapy; if someone wants to be more confident as a public speaker for example, we can use a light trance to get him or her to recall in detail all the characteristics of their favourite speaker. We can then get them to imagine stepping inside that person and feeling how they stand or move when public speaking; hearing their voice from the inside, including their own internal voice; seeing the group they are speaking to; and experiencing how it feels to be confident in that situation. This process can elicit great results and is also used with some sports psychologists who get young hopefuls to model their idols in exactly the same way, to learn or perfect a skill.

Think about all the people you know who have the kind of eating habits you would like. Whenever you come into contact with them, pay special attention to exactly how they behave around food: what they eat, what they leave, and even things like how quickly, or more likely slowly, they eat (slimmer people generally eat more slowly than their fat friends). The more you notice, the more you will begin to notice your own habits and how they differ. This makes slow thinking much easier and it then comes more naturally. At the beginning of the book I said, 'Awareness is curative', and it absolutely is.

Exercise

After a few days or weeks of watching other people and doing your research into how other people make different choices, take it one step further and do this visualization exercise:

- Pick one specific person whom you admire. If there's no one, then create someone in your imagination. Make sure you know exactly how they behave around food and what choices they make.

- Get yourself in a comfortable and fully supported position, turn off all phones or distractions and close your eyes.

- To induce an alpha brain wave state, begin to relax your body. Perhaps start at the top of your head and imagine a smooth golden liquid flowing down the back of your head and into your spine, and as it flows down your spine it branches off through all the nerves sending a message of relaxation to all your muscles. Move gradually at your own pace, down your arms, all around your rib cage and down into your stomach, hips, thighs, knees and eventually, toes. Pay special attention to your breathing. Notice the speed of each breath and how easy it is to breathe without thinking. Notice also that your weight is totally supported and that you can take the weight off your muscles, and your mind.

- As you relax physically, bring an image of this person into your mind's eye, as if you were a fly on the wall watching them. Put them in a situation where you can see them making great, happy, light food choices and they are avoiding sad, heavy foods. Run a movie in your mind's eye and when you have finished a particular meal or food situation, fast forward to another one. Watch until you can predict what they are going to choose to eat/leave before they even do it. Spend as long as you like on this part of the exercise.

- Now rewind the movie and freeze frame on the first shot. Next, imagine you can float inside this person and see through their eyes, feel through their body and hear what they hear, as if you are an invisible guest inside their awareness. Now run the entire movie again from this perspective, even feel them smile when they smile. Feel how comfortable and natural these food choices are from this perspective.

- Run this movie at least twice and then 'save' it so that you can watch it, or recall excerpts of it whenever you want to, even if you do this without thinking. When you can see the movie as a past event, then you are encoding the new maps into your left hemisphere where strategies are created and stored.

· ·

The Magic of Autosuggestion

When you truly convince your unconscious mind of your genuine and deep desire for a healthy, slimmer body, you create a strong *definiteness of purpose*. You have now begun the process of autosuggestion or self-hypnosis, which will change how you think and feel about food for good. Your unconscious will begin to drive your behaviours automatically towards that goal. However, it is important to keep in mind that you are always at the steering wheel! There is no such thing as autopilot when it comes to achieving a goal; you must actively participate in achieving it every day. When you do achieve it, then you can go on to autopilot to stay on track – as long as you install an early warning system!

People are sometimes uncomfortable with the word 'hypnosis'; even the term self-hypnosis can unsettle some people. This is entirely due to a misunderstanding of the concept of being in a suggestive state, or 'trance'. We have explored the fact that you have two minds – a conscious mind and an unconscious one – and that your unconscious contains all the 'data' from every experience you have ever had, which it orders and files to create your beliefs and values and, ultimately, to generate your habitual behaviours. Whether you like it or not, much of that information was gained when you were in a trance, or a hypnotic state.

Many people believe that hypnosis is a form of unconsciousness resembling sleep, but in fact hypnotic subjects are fully awake (even though they may have their eyes closed). They are focusing attention specifically on their internal thoughts, around what they are seeing (in their imagination) or hearing (self-talk or another voice). This 'focused concentration' brings with it a corresponding decrease in peripheral awareness, sometimes to the extent that the individual relaxes deeply physically.

This can enhance the physicality of the experience, but is not essential for 'hypnosis' to take place. In this state of heightened awareness of internal thoughts, we are highly responsive to accepting suggestions. In fact, this happens to you every day in conversation with other people, and you probably aren't even aware of it. It's the basis for almost every marketing strategy ever devised!

Lost in a Trance

Let's look at the occasions in your everyday experience when you may have been in a 'wide-awake' hypnotic state. Have you ever been to a live music concert where the whole audience was totally carried away and immersed in the music? One thing is common to all the really successful bands or performers, and that is the ability to 'trance out' thousands of people at once. A few years ago I went to see David Bowie. It was the best live performance I have ever seen, bar none. He literally had the crowd eating out of his hand – Wembley Stadium was packed to the rafters, and all eyes were focused on one person and what he was saying/singing. More recently I went to see Kylie Minogue, who, with a completely contrasting style, also had the crowd hanging on to her every word.

On both occasions, it was mass hypnosis on a grand scale, and the performers inducing the trance were also totally hypnotized – by their audience. If you've ever been so completely immersed in a book or a TV programme that you block out your surroundings, then you have experienced self-hypnosis, or trance. Have you ever driven somewhere and then wondered how you got there? That's another example of an everyday trance.

In the past, hypnosis has had a bad press. Some of the stage hypnotists who get people to imagine they are famous rock stars and then have them 'perform' to the crowd have been criticized for using the technique. But you must trust your unconscious in that it will *only* allow you to do things, or behave, in a way that is in line with your beliefs. The people who jump around the stage impersonating Tina Turner or Tom Jones are often really quiet types – the reality is that some part of their unconscious sees other more extrovert characters doing things they might like to try, if only they had the 'courage'. By volunteering for stage hypnosis they are giving themselves the chance to be free from their limitations for a few minutes, and to experience something new. That is a conscious choice; they will be fully aware at all times of what is going on, and unless their unconscious is totally in agreement, they will not go along with it.

If you have ever watched a stage hypnotist you will see that he or she gives suggestions to the whole audience and then asks for volunteers to come up on stage. They will only select the people they have seen be compliant with the suggestions given so far, though, and once on stage, the group will be whittled down even further. Those not fully accepting of the process will be thanked and invited to return to their seats. Believe me when I say that no one left on that stage is there for any reason other than wanting to be free of their limitations, if only for a few minutes. After the event they will have full and total recall of exactly what happened and even how they felt about it – they will laugh at themselves as they say, 'It wasn't really me!' but of course, it was totally them! In the modelling exercise in the previous chapter, you are simply generating a trance-like state to create an experience that can induce powerful learning. The more you see yourself doing the things that will make you slim, the more natural they will become. The only limiting factor is your imagination.

As humans we are blessed with the ability to analyze and think, this is largely the job of System 2, or your slow thinking process. This is what sets us apart from animals. Many years ago flea circuses were popular among street entertainers. The fleas would literally jump over a mini object. So how do you train a flea to jump to a certain height? It's easier than you might think. If you were to put a flea in a cup it would of course jump out and be free; but if you put a lid on the cup the flea learns quickly how high to jump without bumping his head. The bad news for the flea is that when you remove the lid, and even if you tip him out of the glass, he remembers that this is the only safe height to jump and forever more will only jump this high. You will have installed a limitation on his ability that he believes is true — even though it isn't. How many limitations do you have, which were imposed by someone else? I have good news — you are not a flea! You can awaken from that particular state and un-hypnotize yourself, freeing you to achieve your potential.

Walking Through Walls

There is a wonderful book called *Hypnotizing Maria* by my very favourite author Richard Bach (author of *Jonathan Livingston Seagull*). It tells the story of a young man called Jamie who goes to a stage hypnotist's show. Jamie volunteers when asked because he thinks it might be fun, although he doubts he can be hypnotized and says as much in a whisper to the hypnotist as he walks on stage. After whittling the volunteers down to just Jamie, the hypnotist invites him to take a walk 'in his mind' down some steps to a beautiful place. Once there, he invites him to open a large wooden door and go through it.

The hypnotist replies that Jamie has created the walls in his own mind and can walk through them simply by believing he can. He tells Jamie, 'You must never be a prisoner of your own limiting self beliefs.' To prove this the hypnotist tells him that he will come into the room with him, take his hand and show him the way out. He walks through the wall behind Jamie, takes his hand, and disappears through the wall in front of them. With a huge concentration of effort Jamie follows him through the wall and back onto the stage...

The process of visualization, combined with emotion and belief, will change the way you think and behave – it will literally overwrite any previous programmes, create brand new neurological pathways and maps and create an unshakable faith in you that you *will* succeed.

Remember that your unconscious is *always* listening: it's like an internal 'Big Brother' who watches everything you do. Your unconscious isn't open to logical thinking in the way that your conscious mind is – it just acts on whatever information it receives – and it doesn't make the same kind of emotional decisions, especially when you are using fast thinking. It has a few golden rules however, and number one is to protect you. That means if you keep telling yourself dieting and exercising are going to be painful, and that you hate them and visualizing how hard it is going to be, then your unconscious will sabotage your efforts in order to protect you from the unpleasant experience.

The flip side to this is that when you begin to hear yourself regularly saying (or thinking) that you are taking more care of your body, that you want to be slimmer because it means being healthier, that you enjoy eating new and different foods, that you enjoy moving your body more, then your unconscious will start to generate behaviours to support these statements.

Combining strong regular visualizations with on-going positive statements will definitely bring you the results you want. A key factor when it comes to visualization is this:

Your unconscious mind cannot tell the difference between reality and imagination.

This means that if you genuinely experience something, or if you imagine you experience something with enough feeling, both are recorded as genuine experiences, and the information from them is stored in exactly the same way in your unconscious 'data files', which dictate your thoughts, beliefs and behaviours.

Imagination Is Reality

Have you ever seen a movie that was so scary that you couldn't get it out of your mind, or a book that contained descriptions or images that actually caused your heart to race? Perhaps you started to sweat or to breathe more heavily? How does this happen? You know consciously it's all make-believe, that none of it is real, don't you? The answer is that you imagine yourself being in that situation and how you would feel, and at that moment it becomes a 'real' experience.

In 1975, a movie came out about a shark that was killing people who were swimming just off the beach. The shark used for filming was made of plastic and rubber – in fact, for most of the shots they didn't even use a full shark model, just the front half because that was all that was in view – and the blood was just sticky, coloured liquid, and yet *Jaws* instilled so much fear in viewers that some left the cinema shaking and could never go in the sea again. In their imaginations, it was *them* in the sea, with a real shark, and it terrified them. Even a snippet of the famous soundtrack is still enough to make some people shudder with genuine fear. Such is the power of the imagination – it changes our 'brain juice'.

This is *good news*, though, because it shows us that we can use our imaginations to create an alternative reality, and when we convince our unconscious of this new reality, it *literally* changes our behaviours to match it. I'm sure you have heard the term 'self-fulfilling prophecy'. This is when people talk about something so much that it actually happens. Usually this refers to a negative state, when people keep talking about and visualizing how they are not going to pass that driving test, not going to do well at that job interview or how their relationship will end… and then when these things happen, they act surprised, but still manage to say, 'I knew that would happen' or 'I saw that one coming!' For many of these people, the *only* reason these things happened was because they were directing their unconscious to *make* it happen.

You don't have to sit and close your eyes to visualize a new outcome. Positive daydreaming is just as effective when you are awake and active. The technical term is 'positive hallucination'. Many people are highly skilled at negative hallucination, and can clearly 'see' what is likely to go wrong in a given situation. As we have learned, this is how negative self-fulfilling prophecies occur. Now with the techniques in this book and your new understanding of how your brain works, you can create a positive self-fulfilling prophecy. Your brain will create your future either based on past assumptions and associations, or new ones. If you want to keep what you have already got, don't change. If you want something different, you must first see yourself achieving it and in doing so, create the neurological pathways that make it inevitable.

•••••••••••••••••••••••••••

Chapter 7

Mind Your Own Business

Here's a thought for you: start minding your own business. By this I mean taking control of your mind to generate your own physical, emotional, mental and spiritual reality.

If you have a garden, or have ever been to a stately home with a beautiful garden, you will know that to keep it looking good takes effort. You can't just plant seeds and expect them to grow into perfect flowers – you must nurture them, clear the weeds from around them, water them and tend them regularly. If you do this you are rewarded with a prize of great beauty, a piece of creation that can be appreciated by all who come into contact with it. On the other hand, have you ever wondered why it is that weeds can grow extremely well with no nurturing or attention whatsoever? What's more, they suck all the nutrients out of the soil so the beautiful plants can't grow there; when beautiful plants do try to poke their lovely heads through the soil, they are quickly strangled and destroyed by the weeds.

Negative thoughts are just like weeds. If left alone, they will multiply and suffocate anything really worth growing. However, when they are pulled out, and more positive thoughts are nurtured, the rewards are immense. If we need water and specialized plant food to help plants grow, then we must need something to help positive thoughts grow.

Many self-help books advocate making statements and reading them out loud, but as you have learnt, words alone, expressed without emotion, are completely worthless. Writing a positive statement, specific to what you want to achieve, *is* a good thing, but you *must combine it with emotion* if you are to activate it. If you want words and statements to become part of your unconscious and remap your brain then you have to emotionalize them, otherwise they are just words.

This exercise takes practice – it needs constant repetition to develop the skill. Remember that Morris Goodman struggled to take his first breath with the respirator, yet within just a few weeks he was breathing completely unaided. You must be persistent, focus deliberately on what you want, and see yourself as having already achieved it. Make sure you do this every day. If Morris can teach himself to breathe, you can surely teach yourself not to eat rubbish foods and not to overeat – I think you can – what do you think?

Using Your Imagination

In the previous chapter you created a visual image of you having achieved your goal. Now we are going to add the words to that image that will create the reality.

If you want to do or achieve something, then it stands to reason that you should identify exactly what you must do to get there. This is a level of understanding accepted by your conscious and your unconscious minds – it's the process of consequence. If you eat too much, the consequence is that you get fat and unhealthy; if you eat less and move more, the consequence is that you get slimmer and healthier.

Your imagination functions on two levels:

- **Previous experiences – Synthetic Imagination** – This organizes or reorganizes already produced old or existing data.

- **New possibilities and realities – Creative Imagination** – This creates new ideas and receives inspiration from sources other than known data. Connects with the sixth sense, both internally and externally, as 'Infinite Intelligence'.

Most, if not almost all, of the time, people function using their Synthetic Imagination. Great achievers, however, function using their Creative Imagination. Alexander Graham Bell and Thomas Edison both used their Creative Imagination to solve many scientific conundrums and bring us things that we take for granted today: the telephone, moving pictures and light bulbs, to name just a few.

Learning to tap into your Creative Imagination through the process of visualization, and attaching intense emotion and desire to your thoughts, is a fundamental skill in achieving something new. Not everyone is skilled at visualization (although it comes quickly with practice) and some people prefer more auditory references instead. That means the pictures must have sounds or words to accompany them. Providing the words generate an emotion, they are hugely powerful, but as you know, without emotion, they are just words.

Exercise

Make a written statement in your journal (visit www.theplacebodiet.co.uk) outlining specifically what you want to achieve and by when, and include what you are prepared to do in exchange. It might look something like this:

'By 1 January next year, I, Janet Thomson, will have achieved a dress size 12. I will be healthier and I will be able to power walk for 4 miles easily without experiencing exhaustion. I will be energized and fit. In exchange, I will eat less, both in portion sizes and in the mindless eating of snacks. I will enjoy moving my body more through regular fast walks and trips to the gym. It's a done deal.'

It's important to include your name: remember *you* are going to be hearing this! Also, note the phrase, '*I will have* achieved' – this is more powerful than '*I will have* gone down *x number of dress sizes.*' You have more positive associations with the word 'achieved' than with 'gone down'.

Now it's your turn: ....

....

....

....

When you are happy with what you have written, read it out loud. You must do this at least twice a day: first thing in the morning (learn it by heart so you can do it in the shower!) and last thing at night. If you do not do this one small thing, then you do not have the desire to change your mind and lose the weight! You are going to have to stay feeling like S.H.I.T. until you opt for something better.

• •

Do this exercise regularly, and your faith in your ability will grow and grow and the kinds of decisions and choices you make around food and activity will change automatically. As you learn more and more about how your body works and handles different foods by reading this book, you will already be deciding what changes you can make to your lifestyle before I even give you the specific guidelines, because you will have a *definiteness of purpose*. You must create a desire for a healthy body that is so strong that not achieving it is not an option. I bet even now, before you have got to the 'food bit', that you can already think of things and ways to change your behaviours so you lose weight; can you?

Anchoring: Take Control of What Triggers Your Behaviours

An anchor is simply something that triggers a specific thought – the exact *same* thought each time the trigger is pulled. It can be an image, a sound, a piece of music or a food. You are being 'anchored' or 'primed' all the time in your daily life. For example, most advertisements try to find something appealing and then anchor it to a specific product as we saw earlier In the McVitie's example. Why do you think so many motorbike adverts show a scantily clad girl writhing all over the bike? It's to anchor sex appeal to the bike. Anchoring is simply a strong form of association between a 'thing' and a feeling. In Chapter 3 you learnt how thoughts become 'things'. And in the 'Your Two Minds' illustration (see *page 46*) you can see that it's a combination of thought and emotion that creates a powerful association, and that becomes a behaviour.

Anchors or triggers can be positive or negative. If you've ever eaten a food that made you sick, then you probably don't ever want to eat it again – that's a negative anchor. Perhaps a piece of music or a place brings back a happy or a sad memory.

For many people food is a powerful anchor. When I was young, whenever I was upset my mum would smile kindly and say, 'Stop crying Janet and you can have a biscuit.' The result was –

I got pretty good at pretending to cry and ate a lot of biscuits. I developed such a sweet tooth that I was the only one of my friends that had fillings. One day at the dentist, I had a root filling that went wrong and I was in the dentist's chair for over two hours screaming. As a child this was a horrific experience, as you can imagine. Eventually the dentist completed the task and made it very clear that if I hadn't eaten so much sugar, I wouldn't have had to have any fillings at all. In one painful instant many of the sweet foods I loved lost their appeal. One neurological map was immediately replaced by another. I do still enjoy the occasional biscuit but I can no longer eat my way through a packet, as I used to do.

Exercise

Choose a food that has contributed to your fatness, e.g. chocolate, crisps, cheese or pies. Then hold it in your hand and stand as naked as possible in front of a mirror, holding it up and showing you and your image the food. Addressing the food say to it, 'You *******[insert angry word of your choice], you did this to me!' If you combine enough painful emotion with the image and the food, you will create an association and an anchor that will change the way you feel about that food. It will lose its appeal.

In my clinic, I once treated a lady who wanted to lose weight for her wedding in a few months. She said she was really struggling to give up some foods that she loved, even though she knew they were 'a sin'. One of these foods was the processed meat stick, 'Peperami'. If you have ever seen the advert for it, you will know that it is given cartoon arms and legs, huge big eyes and a croaky menacing voice. The slogan says 'Peperami — It's a bit of an animal!' as it flings itself, arms and legs waving, across the screen. She worked in an office that had a vending machine that stocked Peperami and told me, 'It calls out to me!' I asked her what specifically it said and she replied, 'Well it just says – eat me I am delicious!' I said, 'That's interesting' and I leapt out of my chair, arms and legs waving, doing a great impression of a Peperami and asked her, 'How would it make you feel if it said, "Come over here you fat cow. I am going to ruin your wedding! I am going to be on your thighs in every single photo – you will see me for years and years in your wedding album and you will always remember how fat you felt in that wedding dress."' She put her hands to her face in horror and said, 'I would want to stamp on it!' We spent the next five minutes visualizing the Peperami calling out to her, saying it was going to ruin her wedding. She even walked across the room, imagining passing the vending machine. The next day I got a great text saying she had not only walked past it, but when no one was looking she made a rude gesture and told it to '**** off' and that it was not invited to the wedding.

This is a great example of how some honest slow thinking can change how you feel about something, and completely rewire your brain, creating new associations, which lead to new habits and behaviours, no will power required.

The following exercise is a classic NLP technique that you can learn to do yourself to great effect.

Creating an Anchor

You need to be in a 'peak' state – a state of intense emotion – to create an anchor. When you are doing this intentionally, as in the following exercises, you need to be able to intensify a thought or association vividly in your mind, be fully associated into it, and then create the anchor at the 'peak' of the experience.

It may take a few minutes of concentration to generate enough emotion to be able to 'set' the anchor. Start to get yourself into the desired state, and when you achieve the maximum level you can create your anchor and then reduce the intensity.

Exercise

Crushing Cravings

If you want to stop desiring chocolate (or any other sweet, fatty or unhealthy food that you crave) you can simply anchor the taste and texture of chocolate to something disgusting. Then, every time you see chocolate, you remember this disgusting taste and not only do you no longer crave it, but it repulses you so much that you just cannot eat it.

1. **Think of a food you crave**, but want to stop wanting (e.g. chocolate).

2. **Think of the worst thing you have ever tasted** – this needs to be something so repulsive that it makes you retch to even think about it. Perhaps you once ate something that made you physically sick? Or maybe you have seen a TV show where celebrities in the jungle forced down something like raw testicles or eyeballs? Think about those foods now. Now add to that some imaginary body fat scraped off the floor of a sauna at the end of the day, mixed in with some pubic hair from a public shower. Mix all these 'flavours' and textures together and imagine how they would taste and how they would smell and feel as if you really did have them in your mouth now. Close your eyes and take a moment to *really* do this, and when the revulsion is at its peak (imagine you really are retching), squeeze the thumb and the index finger of your *left* hand together as you focus on the taste and the slimy, revolting texture.

3. **Create a mind blank by focusing on something different**, like a blue elephant for example, then repeat step two. Do this at least six times

until as soon as you squeeze your left index finger and thumb, you automatically imagine the taste and the smell, and see in your mind's eye the revolting mess and want to retch. You have now created a powerful negative anchor.

4. **Now think about the food you want to stop craving** – get a sense of the taste, texture and smell, and mix those sensations together with the repulsive mixture, so you have, for example, a chocolatey blob of someone else's body fat, a squishy testicle or eyeball and pubic hair mixed together; use your imagination to really blend and combine the two until they are totally linked. Go inside your mouth now and experience the combination of the two things; see what it looks like, feel what it feels like in your mouth. Is it slimey? Perhaps crunchy? How does it smell? Squeeze your left index finger and thumb again once they are totally combined in your imagination, and force yourself to physically swallow when the thought is at its most intense. Blank your mind and think about blue elephants. Repeat this at least six times.

Now test it; have the food in front of you, look at it, use your negative anchor and imagine how revolting it felt and tasted to do the exercise. Remember that now you have put that food behind you.

Some people don't even need to give the food a horrible taste; they just use the worst feeling they have about feeling fat (check out your journal to remind yourself of this exercise). Any strong enough negative association will work, as long as it's genuinely created and accessed.

Every time you see the food you used to crave, squeeze your left index finger and thumb together and remember how violently sick it makes you feel. Use the finger squeeze to recreate it any time that you need to.

....

This technique primes your fast thinking System 1 to react very differently whenever you are exposed to this food. You don't need to rely on the slower thinking System 2 to come up with logical reasons why you should not have it – you just won't want it.

Positive Anchoring

The previous exercise is a good example of how to use a negative anchor to achieve something positive. You can also use a positive experience from a different situation to replicate a feeling of motivation and faith in your ability to achieve something. What feeling would you like to have right now that will help you to believe faithfully that you can change your mind and achieve whatever you want? Perhaps it's something from the list below, or perhaps it's something else:

- Confidence?
- Skill?
- Belief?
- Power?
- Control?
- A sense of achievement?

Decide which of these feelings would be of value to you now, then do the exercise below to associate this feeling with your ability to make the changes you want to make, so that you can lose weight easily.

Exercise

1. **Visualize how you would like to look and feel going about your daily routine differently** – eating differently and moving your body more. Notice how you feel. How strong, on a scale of 1–10, is your belief in your ability to make these changes? (1 is not at all and 10 is absolutely convinced.)

2. **Now think of a time when you had a strong faith in your ability to achieve something that resulted in you actually achieving it.** Perhaps you felt confident or had a sense of achievement when you passed your driving test, or had a successful interview? If you can't remember a time then *create one* in your imagination. Imagine that you totally and utterly nailed it – whatever it was. See yourself, in your mind's eye, looking and feeling strong and indestructible, having achieved something that really meant something. Blend your reality with your Creative Imagination to create a vivid, strong image and feeling. When it really peaks, when you can genuinely manifest the feeling, squeeze the index finger and thumb on your *right* hand together, or if you prefer, make a fist or some other gesture, to anchor that feeling.

3. **Blank your mind** – think of purple giraffes and then repeat step two at least six times.

Now think about all the things you need to do to change the way you think about food and activity. See yourself achieving your goals and all that you desire, see yourself doing specific things differently, such as walking past the vending machine, and as you see these movies of yourself having made the changes and doing things differently, simultaneously fire your positive anchor and remind yourself of how good it feels to achieve something worthwhile. Pay attention to the emotion; are you happy? Proud? Smiling? Confident? In control? Or maybe all of these and more! Enjoy this feeling for a few minutes, then blank your mind and think about purple giraffes. Repeat the process at least six times, each time seeing the movie of your new behaviour and firing that feel-good anchor.

The more you use, or 'stack', an anchor, the stronger it gets. Every time you successfully stop eating *before* you are over-full – i.e. you stop eating when you've had enough – fire that positive anchor off to strengthen it; to acknowledge feeling good about your progress. Every time you do some exercise or activity, fire it off again. You should be firing it off numerous times every day and at the same time seeing yourself *absolutely* achieving your goal. Staying fat is no longer an option – you have absolute *faith* in your ability and it is a *certainty*.

· ·

Your imagination is the control centre for how you change your thoughts and beliefs, and ultimately your behaviour. Remember the quote from the Introduction:

> *'You are free to choose, but you are not free*
> *from the consequence of that choice.'*

Mirror Neurons

One of the exciting developments in neuroscience over recent years has been the discovery and understanding of mirror neurons. As the name implies, these neurons become active through the process of observing others. We have all seen someone stub their toe have and winced in associated pain, or recoiled and held our own hand when someone shows us a bad cut on their hand. This ability to instinctively and unconsciously react to others is down to our mirror neurons.

The discovery of mirror neurons was almost accidental. In the early 1990s, Italian researchers implanted electrodes in the brains of several macaque monkeys to study their brain activity during different motor actions, including reaching for and holding food. One day, as a researcher reached for his own food, he noticed neurons begin to fire in the monkeys' premotor cortex—the same area that showed activity when the animals made a similar hand movement themselves. How could this be happening when the monkeys were sitting still and merely watching him? Some part of their brains were recognizing an action similar to their own and they were having the same neurological response. They were externally inactive i.e. not moving or reaching for food, but neurologically they were internally mirroring what they saw.

Through mirroring you can create new neurological pathways and maps without doing anything. This is why it is so important to surround yourself with people who do what you want to do and behave as you want to behave. Many studies have shown that the chances of children smoking are drastically increased if they see their parents smoke, and if the parents are obese they are highly likely to become obese. The children learn new patterns and create them unconsciously through mirroring. In the early chapters about brain structure and the concept of neuroplasticity, we learned that up until the end of adolescence our brains are especially plastic. This is when we are most influenced by the actions of others. This explains a lot of adolescent behaviour! Have you ever heard a parent say to a child, 'Do what I say, not what I do!' The problem is the child will not do what the adult says, they will do what they see them do.

Before the discovery of mirror neurons, scientists generally believed that our brains used logical thought processes to interpret and predict other people's actions, and rationalize them by comparing them to our own. However new research demonstrates it's not a thought, but a feeling, that is activated when mirror neurons fire. Have you ever noticed yourself smiling just because other people are smiling around you, without any conscious thinking or words being spoken? And we know from earlier in the book that the body talks to the mind, in this case we mirror other people's facial muscles and the body sends that message to the brain which says, 'I'm smiling – I must feel good!' and generates the neurochemistry to feel good. You do not need to know the reason behind anyone else's smile – it's a non-cognitive exchange of information based purely on observation. People around you may influence you more than you think! Just this week on Facebook, a friend posted a clip that was going viral, of a woman on the London Underground looking at something on her phone that was really making her laugh, not just giggle, but a real belly laugh. Pretty soon all the people around her started to laugh, even though they had no idea what she was finding so funny. Some people were almost hysterical; it was a perfect example of the power of mirror neurons.

Potentially, it's easy to adopt someone else's habits, especially if there are a group of people doing the same thing. Our early ancestors who lived as hunter gatherers increased their chances of survival when they lived as a group, as they could combine collective abilities to hunt, gather food that was safe to eat, build effective shelter and so on. Imagine if every single person had to learn all that for themselves or had to have it all explained to them cognitively. By watching and observing each other, information was exchanged and mirrored. Even language is thought to have evolved through a process using mirror neurons. Many hand gestures use the same neural brain circuits as some complex lip-and-tongue movements used during speech. It's proposed that hand gestures came first and the associated sounds were the basis for early language.

So what has this got to do with weight loss? Have you ever been at a social gathering or maybe at the office when someone brings the cakes in and you resolved not to have anything? Then you see someone else enjoying the cake and smiling. The drive to do the same is almost instant and all your resolve goes out of the window. Mirror neurons are involved in that process. They want you to get that same feeling that you are seeing in someone else and if you saw what they did that made them smile, the answer is obvious – do that! Mirror neurons are not neurologically the same process as when we are using System 1 (fast thinking) because the whole point is, you are not actually thinking. Observation is the cue; it's a whole different neurological circuit, but the speed of action is exactly the same.

I have good news: because your brain can't tell the difference between an imagined image and a real one, when you create a strong image of you as you want to be (as the journal exercises and I have been guiding you to do throughout), then your mirror neurons will fire whenever you see 'you' in the future, looking happy while doing the things that made you slim. All of the exercises in this programme are based on sound neuroscience principles and now you really know how to change your mind and transform your body. There is a lot more to come as well.

IMPORTANT NOTE

Revisit all the visualization exercises in your journal and remind yourself to create a strong image of 'you' in the future and daydream about her/him many times through the day. Have her/him pop into your mind regularly, especially if it is a vision, but even just a 'sense' of you even if you can't yet see you, will have the same effect. Remember – everything we do is to get a feeling. Imagining how it feels to be happy and free from dieting, and naturally making great food choices, is an important part of the process of creating new neurological circuits.

Chapter 8

Attitude or 'Fat-titude'?

I said earlier in the book that I don't know how long you've been fat, other than it's been too long, otherwise you wouldn't be reading this book. The reason for your fatness has been in your attitude – or should I say your 'fat-titude' towards food, activity, and ultimately your body, and how you feel about yourself? How much you value yourself is vital in determining how much care you take of yourself. The L'Oréal adverts don't use the phrase 'Because you're worth it!' for nothing! It all comes down to your attitude.

Your attitude is ultimately the means by which you compile, and then apply, what you experience through a process of thinking. If each individual thought is a piece of your jigsaw puzzle, your attitude is the complete image it creates. It's what you see on a daily basis when you put it all together. Your thoughts create your image, and that's both a metaphor and a reality!!!

Napoleon Hill believed that it is your consistent, repetitive thoughts that form your attitude – they determine who you are and what you can achieve. He said: 'All thoughts which have been emotionalized and mixed with faith begin immediately to translate themselves into their physical equivalent.'

Hill demonstrated the power of positive thinking to create a positive mental attitude when a traumatic event happened in his own life. After Hill's wife gave birth to a son, the doctor came into the waiting room and asked Hill to prepare himself for a shock. He told him that his son had been born without ears and would never be able to hear – he would be a deaf-mute. Hill immediately told the doctor that he would find a way to enable his son to hear. For the next decade he devoted a huge amount of time to working with his son, trying to get him to respond to sound. He was successful and as a direct result of his unrelenting efforts, and his absolute faith in his ability to find a way, the child attained a level of functional hearing. He attended a regular school and was far from being a mute – his speech was normal.

When he was 25, Hill's son went to see a leading ear specialist in New York. After conducting a series of x-rays and examinations, the consultant stated that although he could see no evidence of any form of physical hearing equipment, the tests had confirmed that the young man had 65 per cent of the normal hearing ability. It was completely inexplicable and the doctor declared it a 'miracle'. The consultant also said he thought that, without a doubt, the psychological directives Hill had consistently given his son over the years had somehow activated a process through the boy's unconscious whereby he adapted and influenced nature to be able to improvise a reorganization of his nervous system. This subsequently connected his brain with the inner walls of the skull and enabled him to hear through a process that later became known as 'bone conduction'.

You Can Do the Impossible at Once, but Miracles Take a Little Longer

The consistently positive attitude and self-belief demonstrated by both Napoleon Hill and Morris Goodman achieved the impossible. Don't tell me you can't imagine yourself not eating chocolate, cakes, crisps, cheese, or whatever else you put in your mouth when you are not hungry, because I don't buy it. Nor should you (the thought, not the chocolate; come to think of it, don't buy the thought or the chocolate!).

If you were to interview 100 of the world's top achievers from a variety of backgrounds and disciplines – e.g. sportspeople, business people, teachers, authors, film producers and politicians – you would find a common denominator. And that common denominator is a positive attitude. On the other hand, if you were to interview 100 non-achievers from the same disciplines or backgrounds, you would also find a common denominator: negativity. The latter would probably be in the form of blaming others, or the circumstances, or just being unlucky, or in the wrong place at the wrong time or missing the boat. The reality is that achievers experience bad luck and misfortune as often as anyone else, they just handle it differently. They chalk it up to experience and move on. If you have 'failed' on a previous 'diet' then stop blaming the diet and get over it. You learnt what doesn't work and that's a valuable lesson because you don't have to waste your time doing it anymore.

Over the years I have heard just about every excuse in the book for people's failure to lose weight. Here are just a few of the more common ones:

- I don't have time
- My husband/wife/partner won't eat healthy food

- It was Christmas/a birthday/a holiday that made me put on 3kg (7lbs)
- It's because of my job
- Obesity runs in the family
- I don't like fruit and vegetables.

The list goes on and on. What would you add? Who or what do you blame for your fatness?

If you use this kind of language, then your fat-titude stinks! You are using 'stinking thinking' and you need to *stop* and start thinking like a slim person – that is, a *happy* slim person. If you see slim people as sad and miserable because they can't stuff their faces, then that's a good thought to change right away! When you think about slim people, think about happy, healthy, slim (not skinny) people. After all, there are unhappy people of all shapes and sizes! Let's just focus on the positive ones.

When your attitude is negative, and you repeatedly make excuses for why you are fat, and why you can't get slim, you are justifying your behaviours and creating a powerful belief that will direct your unconscious toward maintaining that fatness. Everything you have learnt so far about your thoughts, and the effects of your thoughts, will have taught you that.

Just as a quick check-in, on a scale of 1–10, with 10 being absolute certainty and 1 no chance, how do you rate the likelihood of you actually making the changes we have been talking about? If you do apply them, when you have got all the information you need from the colour-code system – you will lose weight; it's as simple as that. Think of this part of the programme as learning how to use a computer. The colour-code system, when combined with all you have learnt about using the hardware, will create a new super-computer in your mind that has been completely cleaned up and updated, and is free from previous embedded viruses and electronic infections.

Exercise

If you want to be slim, you must genuinely and faithfully change your attitude towards your health and your body.

Let me ask you a personal question – where do you live? Send me the answer now, telepathically.

If you gave me a physical address, that's not where you live; that is your second home. Your address is where your first home is geographically located, but you live in your body.

Write down the answers to these questions (in your journal) as if you were preparing the brochure for a house sale: would it be in need of updating/ refurbishing or perhaps full refurbishment?

Description of outside ....

....

Description of inside ....

....

Your Body Is Your Home

There is a very special and unique part of you, perhaps deep, deep within, that was created *before* you came into physical life – long before you took your first breath. Maybe you refer to this part of you as your 'soul', or your 'spirit'? Whichever phrase you use, this is your absolute essence, the source of who you truly are.

I believe that not only did this part of you exist before you were born, but that it will continue in some sense after your physical body is gone. Whatever *you* believe, know this for sure: there is a part of you that is not physical.

This special part of you – I will call it your spirit (but you may refer to it by any name, such as your soul) – when connected to your physical body, gave you, and still gives you, life. What have you given it back? In return for these gifts, what do you give your spiritual essence? Unlike your physical body, it doesn't live off food and water – it lives and grows, or shrivels and rots, based on the quality of your thoughts and your attitude towards the precious gift of life. How well do you look after the mystical and magical part of you?

There are many ways to look after it. The first and most important is to give it a nice, safe, clean place to live – that's your body. For the first few years of your life, this is the responsibility of your parents, but it has long since been your responsibility. You must accept that responsibility with a sense of gratitude, sincere commitment and responsibility. You can honour your spiritual essence by simply giving it a good home.

If you moved into a new house of the bricks and mortar kind, and it was a mess – with broken windows, crumbling walls, and ceilings that looked like they were about to collapse – and all of this was visible from the *outside*, what would you do? If you would slob out and accept it and do nothing, then what are you doing reading this book? I don't think that's the kind of person you are. Most people who are reading this are much more proactive – they would not tolerate that kind of lifestyle. They genuinely want better things from life. They would refurbish and redecorate – or if that wasn't possible, they would move house. Would you?

Magnetic Attraction

Your mental attitude not only affects your body, it affects every single aspect of your life, including who is in it. Positive people attract positive people; they can't and don't tolerate being around negative people. Take a look at who you spend the most time with. I once heard that you are likely to earn no more than the average income of your five closest friends. *Who* you spend your time with directly affects your attitude, because your unconscious mind is continually processing their shared experiences as well as your own. And because like attracts like (remember how your unconscious likes things that are the same), it's as easy to be drawn to people who have the same weaknesses as you as it is to those who have the same strengths. Having learned all about mirror neurons this makes a lot of sense, so keep it in mind.

I am not suggesting that you ditch any fat friends! But if you do spend a lot of time around people with poor eating habits then you must begin to protect yourself from their language and their behaviours. Create for yourself an invisible set of earmuffs that you can put on whenever they are moaning about this or that. Stop that information from getting through to your ears and create an invisible set of blinds for your eyes, so you can't visually process or associate with their continual 'fat habits'. If you do see them or hear them then it's with new eyes and ears that allows you to associate them with massive pain.

Creating a Strong Mental Attitude

Your mental attitude is *completely* under your influence and control. You simply can't blame anyone else – whatever your situation. You only have to hear the story of Viktor Frankl to appreciate this. Frankl was a prominent and highly esteemed Austrian neurologist who, along with his wife and parents, was captured by the Nazis and deported to a concentration camp in 1942. He continued his work within the camps and prevented countless suicides. His wife was transferred to another camp, where she perished, as did both his parents, but still Frankl continued his work and became even more devoted to helping others. In 1945 the Americans liberated the camp he was in. As a result of his own hideous experiences and suffering in the camp — and that of others — he discovered that even suffering has a meaning. He went on to write *Man's Search for Meaning*, which is an amazing and inspiring story of how a positive attitude can overcome literally any situation.

A strong, positive mental attitude generates inspiration: it puts your sixth sense in touch with God, 'Infinite Intelligence', the 'ether' or the universe. Whatever your belief is, whichever word you use, it's the space that is within you and around you that carries information within it and through itself, and it is a source of power that you can access. You have your own internal receiver and transmitter, and your attitude is what tunes you in — or out — of the right frequency. When you are tuned in, and have a positive mental attitude, you can frame every experience as a potentially beneficial one, even if it doesn't seem like one at the time.

Recently, I was loading my car in preparation for a training seminar with a group of weight-loss clients. It was pouring with rain. A guy who I had never met or seen before walked past me and had a right old moan about the weather, fully expecting me to join in with his negativity. He looked at me, waiting for a response, and I replied, 'Yes, but it's lovely for the ducks!' Completely baffled by my lack of negativity, the man stomped off. It was clear that he was used to being around people who feed his negativity in order to justify it. The ducks and I, however, were quite happy.

Having a negative attitude is a bit like getting sunburned on a cloudy day – you don't realize how harmful it is until it's too late. As Thomas Jefferson said: 'Nothing can stop the man with the right mental attitude from achieving his goal; nothing on Earth can help the man with the wrong mental attitude.' A positive mind keeps itself busy looking for the potential good in *every* situation. If you are going to a birthday party and see this as an excuse or a reason to 'go off the diet', you could instead view it as an opportunity for you to learn how to have a great time without getting fatter. This is a skill that will no doubt come in very handy on countless occasions once you have mastered it!

Exercise

Here are the steps to follow for creating a strong mental attitude: As you read each one give yourself a mark out of 10 for each, with 10 being top marks and 1 being very poor. Make a note in your journal of your scores and then adjust these over time as you feel yourself changing more and more.

- **First, you must create a strong and intense desire for what you want to achieve.** This desire must become a passion, an absolute *must have.* /10

- **Next, you must identify the thoughts and behaviours that have kept you from achieving this goal.** You need to know what you have to *stop* doing before you can *start* doing something else, otherwise you are giving yourself mixed messages. If you are working on your computer and you want to delete a paragraph, you have to find the exact paragraph and highlight it before you can delete it. You need to acknowledge what you are deleting and be prepared to let it go in exchange for having something much better. /10

- **You must generate a clear, visible image or representation of 'you' as already having achieved your goal,** and then generate powerful, positive emotions when you see it. This visualization must be repeated intentionally at least twice daily. /10

- **You must add words or statements to that goal**, and you must repeat them out loud with passion and belief to generate absolute faith and to change your 'brain juice'. You must do this at least twice a day, with your visualizations. When you look at your new image and talk to 'you' with positive language and affirmations, you will engage your mirror neurons, strengthening new neurological circuits and activating your neurological motivation and pleasure centres. /10

- **You must, through the process of positive self-talk, autosuggestion or self-hypnosis, constantly feed yourself positive statements** and directives to maintain healthy 'brain juice', not just when you are visualizing 'you', but all the time. You are never not listening and never not reacting to what you are saying, so choose your words carefully. How you speak to yourself, above all else, determines your destiny. /10

- **You must regularly associate with like-minded people who have already achieved, or are achieving, the same or similar goals.** The sense of belonging to a group is important because it creates a feeling of safety. This is a natural survival instinct based on hunter-gatherers being safer in groups. It can also positively affect 'brain juice'. Make sure you have some positive and encouraging communication every day. Just observing people who already do what you want to do, or have what you would like to have, will activate your mirror neurons. /10

- **You must continue to read and/or listen to audio recordings that will feed your mind with positive thoughts and suggestions.** Aim to do this for at least 15 minutes a day. This is easy to do because most of us have MP3 players on our phones, or CD players in the car. Put something positive on when you are getting dressed in the morning, or listen to it in the car or on the train, instead of putting on the TV and watching depressing news. If you go for a walk, put some headphones on and feed your mind positive information and stories. Start the day with a positive *mental* breakfast as well as a nutritious food one. You can access some free audio downloads and a 10-step guide to 'Change Your Mind' on my therapy website www.powertochange.me.uk, as well as the free, first audio lesson on www.theplacebodiet.co.uk. The recommended reading list at the end of this book is also a great resource. /10

- **You must develop knowledge and skills that will make achieving your goals easier.** In this case, the nutrition and 'how your body works' sections of this book will do this, and the colour-code system puts it all into practice, but read and reread the entire book over and over. This book will be at its most powerful when you are reading sections of it for the second or maybe the third time. When you find you are already thinking ahead to what's coming next, you've got it! Remember, this is *not* a novel – you must read it all the way through, slowly and thoughtfully, and then do it again. And maybe again! It's a resource, and along with the audio downloads from the website, it forms the basis of *all you need to change.* /10

....

Chapter 9

The Habit Loop

Much of what you have learned in this programme explains how neurological maps are formed to create behaviours or responses that you do automatically, without thinking. The common word for this is, of course, a 'habit'. In this chapter we are going to learn more about how habits are formed, and a practical model for how to change them. This chapter will become even more relevant after you have read the nutrition section and the colour-code system. Then, you'll be able to revisit the exercises here to learn how to change food preferences while still loving your food and getting comfort form it!

The basic premise for NLP (Neuro-Linguistic Programming), which was created by Richard Bandler and John Grinder, is the study of what works in human behaviour. Most psychological therapies pay great attention to what is wrong with someone, the things they do that make them feel bad. NLP focuses on what people who don't have the problem do. They then model these kinds of behaviours and teach them to the people with the problem. If someone already knows how to do something that would be useful for you, then model him or her and do what they do. When we use mirror neurons we are, to some extent, modelling people subconsciously, but with NLP there is a deliberate set of Instructions to follow to change how you think and make that change deliberate and conscious. If you have a spider phobia and you see a spider, then right on cue, you will probably distort the image of the spider you can see and replace it with a much bigger, fiercer, Jurassic-Park-style version. It's not the spider you can actually see that you are afraid of; it's the subsequent picture (or movie) that you create in your mind of the giant man-eating spider that scares you. As soon as you get the cue (which may even just be someone talking about spiders), your neural circuitry kicks in for a conditioned response. Although this isn't technically a habit, in principle the neurology is very similar, in that there's a cue or a trigger, and a response. The reason for the response is the reward you get by removing yourself from the threat; the fear goes away and you feel better. When you see the structure of a habit loop you will see the similarities. In therapy we know (using NLP and other techniques) how to collapse a phobic reaction and these same techniques can be equally efficient in changing a habit loop.

How Habit Loops Are Created

There are essentially three steps to creating a habit loop and each is important to understand. You cannot break a habit, but you can change it.

One of the leading experts in the study of habit is Charles Duhigg whose excellent book, *The Power Of Habit*, inspired me to create new techniques for changing behaviour. The book also helped me to understand more clearly why so many of the techniques I was already using in my programmes (in particular visualization) worked so well. It was where I first saw the model of a habit loop.

Step 1: The Cue

This is something that triggers a particular automatic behaviour. In smokers, for example, it may be always having a cigarette with the first coffee of the day. It may be that whenever you hear the music of a particular TV programme you like, you automatically put the kettle on and settle down to watch it with a cup of tea. Cues come in many forms and can be anything from time, to a sound or even a smell.

Step 2: The Behaviour

This is what you do in response to the cue. In the above examples it's smoking or drinking tea.

Step 3: The Reward

You associate pleasure with doing the behaviour, which confirms in your mind you made the right choice, thus reinforcing the neurological map. A reward may be an emotion or a feeling, a taste, something tangible or anything at all that helps you either avoid pain or achieve pleasure.

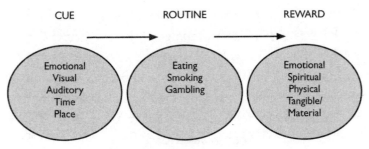

The Process of Cues, Routines and Rewards

How Habits Work

Habits work by allowing our brain to 'chunk down' learnt maps so that our brain is free to concentrate on other things. As we noted early in the book, without habits the amount of daily activities necessary to survive would be overwhelming; every day at work would be like your first day; cooking, cleaning your teeth, literally everything would be done as if for the first time.

Basic training teaches military personnel exactly how to react in a given situation when they might not have time to think and might be suffering from mental and physical fatigue. Airline pilots are trained to react in specific ways if there's a mechanical problem. Athletes train themselves to react to the sound of the starting pistol. Companies install (deliberately or by default) corporate habits that can either enhance or inhibit the company's performance. Parents are taught that if they want their baby to sleep they need to create a bedtime routine and stick to it. Put simply, we need habits.

The problem is that many of our habits were created without our permission.

Eugene Pauly

Eugene Pauly taught scientists much of what is now known about habits and how they become installed. As an adult Eugene suffered from viral encephalitis, which had a dramatic effect on his brain. Against all the odds, he astonished doctors by recovering physically and learning to swallow, talk and walk again. People who met him, who had not known him before the illness, might not have noticed anything at all was wrong.

Although he recovered his physicality, his short-term memory was severely impaired. He could remember in detail things that had happened before the illness, but nothing afterwards. Doctors and nurses had to reintroduce themselves to him even if they had only left him for a few minutes. He would get up in the morning and make himself breakfast. Then he would go back to bed. He would forget he had got up and get up again and make breakfast.

His consultant, Larry Squires, had spent decades studying the 'neuroanatomy of memory' and worked with Eugene for many years. Through observing how Eugene functioned, Squires would finally understand how and where in the brain habits are formed.

Once Eugene was physically well enough, he and his wife moved to a new house to be nearer family. Doctors would visit Eugene in his home to see how he was doing. On one visit he was asked to sketch a layout of the house, but he could not remember where the rooms were. Then he got up, went to the bathroom and returned to the lounge. He had no cognitive memory of which room was where, yet he had learnt where to go to the bathroom and how to get back.

On doctor's advice his wife took him for a walk twice per day, around the area close to their home, but they emphasized she must go with him to avoid him getting lost. One day when she had turned her back, she found he had left the house by himself. She was frantic and ran up and down neighbouring streets looking for him. When she went back to call the police he was sitting on the sofa – against all predictions he had somehow found his way home. He couldn't communicate where he had been, as he didn't remember leaving, but he had brought back some pinecones from the route, as they had done numerous times before. Despite her best efforts to stop him, he began frequently going out by himself, but he always came home; eventually she just let him go for a walk whenever he wanted. He often brought back souvenirs such as the pinecones, and once brought back a puppy! It was clear that he had been unconsciously absorbing new information about the route and using this information to form habits. His new learnt cues were visual; when he saw a certain building or a post box he was prompted to make the correct turn; even though he had no conscious idea he was choosing the right way to go.

Consistent Cues and Triggers

Think about putting your key in your front door. If you have lived in the same place for a while, chances are you can do it just as well in the dark. You see the door (the cue), you get out your key and put it in the slot and the door opens (reward). There will be almost no brain activity in you performing this task after you have done it many times, as it has become a habit; yet when you first did it there would have been a lot more neurological activity.

The cue or trigger that initiates a habit can be anything, but it must be consistent; this is why all chain establishments, such as McDonald's or Starbucks, look the same all over the world. All McDonald's fries are prepared and cooked in such a way that they dissolve in your mouth the minute they touch your tongue to give you an immediate 'hit' or reward, lighting up the pleasure centres in your brain. After a time you don't even need to see a McDonald's sign, just the thought of the chip is enough of a cue to start a craving for the loop.

The Power of Positive Association

It's important to revisit the premise of advertising campaigns here. The company obviously wants you to buy their product or service. We have already learnt how we are primed by associations (such as the kittens in the McVitie's advert) and once primed, these images or situations become a cue for a behaviour that becomes a habit. If you don't have a positive association with the behaviour triggered by the cue, a habit cannot be created, that's why positive priming is so important. The behaviour the companies want from you is that you make a purchase and, in the case of the biscuits, ideally not just once. They want it to become your automatic response; they want to programme your brain for you. Scared? You should be. If you eat a biscuit let it be because you are making a choice to do so, not because of a marketing strategy designed to eliminate all other choices.

Studies of successful weight-loss participants has shown that when starting a new exercise regime, you are more likely to stick to it if you can build in a specific cue, and associate a reward with going to the gym. That cue might be as simple as putting your trainers or workout bag on the front seat of your car instead of in the boot, so that when you finish work they are a reminder. The reward might be something tangible like finishing your session by relaxing in the steam room or sauna, or planning some other activity you enjoy for the evening, watching a movie, meeting friends or anything that makes you feel good that doesn't involve food.

In my own clubs I saw this again and again: the people who attended on the same days each week invariably attended a lot more and got better results than those who just came randomly whenever they had time. They made attendance a habit. Even those who started out with the best intentions dropped off relatively quickly without the routine. The successful members rarely missed a session because it was a habit and the compound effect of regular exercise (more about this coming up soon!) paid dividends in terms of the amount of weight they lost. We have learnt the brain likes us to make our decision-making as easy as possible. If you pre-decide that you will not eat cake for example, when you are faced with a cake you don't have to have an internal discussion, listen to both sides of the argument, and then either eat or not eat it (most likely eat it). If you pre-decide it's not an option, it's much easier. I am a non-smoker, so if someone offered me a cigarette I would say, 'No thanks – I don't smoke'. That's a pretty powerful non-negotiable position. However, if I said, 'No thanks – I am trying to give up'. Then two things will probably happen: firstly my mirror neurons will watch and record the pleasure the smoker gets from their cigarette, and secondly I will start an internal justification as to the benefits, or otherwise, of stopping something that gave me so much pleasure. It's easy to lose resolve and have the cigarette. How many times have you said to an offer of a fattening or heavy food, 'No thanks – I am on a diet'? And the person offering you the food said, 'Go on – just one won't hurt' or something like, 'It's OK, this ice cream is calorie free after 7 p.m.!'? If you do a quick mental check, my guess is the person saying those things to you is a failed dieter. You have to make no, mean no. You can do this by deconstructing the habit loop and disassociating the reward with the current behaviour, in this case the specific food. This eliminates the need for willpower. No means no because you genuinely don't want whatever is being offered.

Identifying Cues, Behaviours and Rewards, and Installing New Habits

A few years ago I saw a friend I hadn't seen for a long time; he had lost almost four stone. I asked him how he did it and he replied, 'By becoming a miserable bast***, I just stopped going out every Friday and Saturday night'. No prizes for guessing that within a few months he was piling the weight back on, and more besides. You have to learn how to keep the things that give you pleasure, in this case going out, and make the choices that allow you to still lose weight. People are often surprised that I eat out as often as I do, a necessity from working away so much. However, I follow the colour-code system guidelines (*see Chapter 14*) whether I am at home or out. It's easy to do and I have plenty of delicious foods to choose from. Going out may be trickier than staying at home and choosing consciously to make something super healthy to boost your metabolism, but it's easy when following the guidelines becomes a habit.

The following exercise (printed in full in your journal) will allow you to identify cues, behaviours and rewards. You cannot break a habit if you are going to be exposed to the same cues, but you *can* change your response to the cue. Remember the Peperami example? I couldn't remove the vending machine from her workplace but I could change her reaction to it and make sure she got more pleasure from not eating one, than she ever got from eating one. This exercise, combined with the other exercises in the programme, will allow you to create a new habit or behaviour in response to cues. In particular the 'Crushing Cravings' exercise (*see page 114*) can be helpful in removing old associations with foods, and creating new positive anchors for new ones.

Exercise

• In column 1 list the 'heavy' foods that have literally made you heavy.

• In column 2 list where/when you eat them. Think about why you go for the same thing each time – what is the cue?

- In column 3 list the reward; is it emotional, physical or something else? Even if it is as simple as relieving boredom, that's a strong enough reward to generate a habit.

- I have added a 4th column to the traditional model, as if you habitually have ice cream when you go out for a meal, but rarely go out for a meal, it doesn't necessarily have to be changed. Even slim people eat ice cream sometimes! The foods you want to pay most attention to are the ones that you eat most often.

FOOD	CUE	REWARD	FREQUENCY
Peperami	See the vending machine	Enjoy taste	Daily

When you have identified your cues, it's time to think about what you could do or eat instead. It may be that you genuinely need to eat. If you are eating for comfort or to replace a negative feeling, the behaviour you replace the food with needs to be non-food related. What you must realize is that the behaviour is generating a feeling or a reward, so in order to give it up, you must do something else instead that also brings a reward. This is where so many diets fail, you just have to stop eating food you like with no real alternative that brings the same pleasure and so, unsurprisingly, you self-sabotage. You know well enough by now that you are programmed to avoid pain and achieve pleasure. This is the basis of all habits.

When you have identified the foods and their cues, complete the following table. If you are looking to replace heavy food with lighter options that are equally delicious, you may want to revisit this table after you have learnt how to use the super simple colour-code system (coming up in Chapter 14). If you are replacing a food that you eat for an emotional hit, then you can complete the table now and start thinking about other things you can do that make you feel good.

FOOD	CUE	NEW HABIT/ BEHAVIOUR	REWARD
Peperami	See the vending machine	Talk back to Peperami and walk past smiling	Feel empowered and happy

The Power of Visualization

When installing new habits it's important to do more than just write them down here. Revisit the practical exercises (and use the guided meditations if you are also following the Placebo Diet at Home online programme) to imprint a new map. If you are still sceptical about the power of visualization exercises, consider the amazing true story behind Michael Phelps's 200-metre butterfly swim final at the 2008 Beijing Olympics.:

> As soon as he entered the water, Phelps knew that something was wrong. His goggles were leaking, and as he powered through the water they gradually filled up until he was unable to see either the lines along the bottom of the pool or the markings indicating the approaching wall. He was 'swimming blind'. But Phelps was able to remain calm, as he and his coach had worked on a programme

of visualization exercises in which Phelps mentally rehearsed every stroke of every race. This meant that he could go with what he knew rather than what he could see, and he knew exactly how many strokes he would need to hit the final wall. He anticipated the final, huge stroke and reached out to touch the wall, and removed his goggles to discover that not only had he won the race, but he had set a new world record. His pattern of habits had made him the best in the world.

You may be happy to know that you don't have to swim an Olympic final to reach your goal. But you do have to use some of the same techniques Phelps used to reach his own goal. Each chapter has built on the one before, and the programme has been carefully researched and designed so that each step takes you closer towards your goal of living in a healthy body.

Small changes in habits might seem insignificant but the compound effect can be enormous. Conventional medical studies have repeatedly advocated a complete change of lifestyle for obese patients. However, I know from my own experience and from the vast amount of research I did during my own studies that *much* more often than not, people just cannot sustain a strict new regime. I mentioned earlier my own study into the effects of food recording, and how when my members wrote down what they ate, they automatically lost weight. In 2009, a group of health researchers at the University of North Texas asked 1,600 obese patients to record everything they ate for at least one day per week. Unsurprisingly there was an unwillingness to comply, however some individuals got into the habit of food recording every day, not just for one. They became aware of their own eating patterns, for example some noticed that they had an unhealthy snack when they got peckish every morning at work at around 11 a.m.. They automatically started preparing for this by taking fruit to eat instead. The cue was still the same but the food changed and they got the same reward, i.e. satisfied appetite. They were not told to make this change. It was purely because they became aware (there's that word again) of a behaviour that wasn't serving them, so they instinctively changed it. Pretty soon the new habit had totally replaced the old. It might seem like a tiny change, but those who kept journals lost over twice as much weight as those who did not. Previously they were like the frog ('this one won't hurt'), but when they removed the food, the compound effect was significant.

Before we leave this chapter, let's take a last look at the concept of willpower.

A few years ago I was writing for a national slimming magazine, and early one January received a reader's letter to answer, which went something like this, 'Please help me – over Christmas I lost my willpower and gained 7lbs! I just could not stop eating the sweets and chocolates on the tree. Every time they got low I just replaced them as the tree looked bare without them, and then I ate those too!'

My reply went like this: 'Firstly, you must be brutally honest with yourself. You did not lose your will power – you can lose your car keys because they are a 'thing' but willpower is a process of exerting choice. You can't lose it. You simply made bad choices and paid the price. All the time you are justifying a behaviour by blaming it on something that you think you can lose whenever it suits you to, you are doomed to fail. You must accept that there is a consequence when you continually put chocolate in your mouth, day after day. The consequence is that you get fat. It's your fault.

*When you have admitted that, you become aware and accept that
you need to learn techniques to help you make better choices. This
combination of awareness and honesty will be your springboard
for success.' I was pretty pleased with that response but the editor
called me immediately upon receiving it and said she could not
possibly print something so blunt. Where she used the word blunt
I would use the word honest, a professional difference that led to
me resigning. Without honesty and an acceptance that to achieve
a different outcome something needs to change, you get what
you have always had. They printed a much-edited, soft and fluffy
version of my response, which I suspect was no help at all.*

Look Who's Talking!

I have mentioned your 'internal voice' a few times throughout the
book. That was to 'prime' you for this section. Your internal dialogue,
above all else, influences what you do. As with all the sections of this
book, I have researched the best teachers so that I can bring you
the very best of the best information available on each subject. For
me, the person who best explains the concept of internal voice is
Michael A. Singer whose beautiful book, *The Untethered Soul* (which
works even better when listened to as an audio book), elegantly
takes you through the process of what it is and how to change it.

Your internal voice is simply the language of conscious
thought, presented as internal dialogue.

We need our internal dialogue to make sense of everything
around us; otherwise we would just exist in a world full of
meaningless 'stuff'. Look at these two examples of the internal
dialogue of a person sitting under a tree. The exact same situation
but completely different internal representation:

- 'There's a lovely tree; it's just like the one in my garden that I love to sit underneath. Oh and there's a puppy! How cute, he reminds me of Sandy the dog I had as a child, I loved that dog!'

- 'There's a lovely tree; it's just like the one in my garden I used to sit under when I wasn't so busy. Oh and there's a puppy, he looks dangerous and reminds me of when I got bitten by a dog as a child.'

Neither dialogue changes the fact that there's a tree and a puppy; but they do change the way you react to them. Either way your dialogue is bringing the world around you into your own personal reality. You internal dialogue manipulates what you see to make it fit your map of the world.

> *'Your internal voice is the narrator of*
> *your life – but it is not your life.'*
> MICHAEL SINGER

You gave your internal voice a very important job i.e. 'look after me, keep me safe, make me happy and successful'. Once you did that, you set in motion a life's work for your internal voice, constantly challenging everything you see, feel or hear so that you can strive to be safe, happy and successful. Once instructed, your internal voice began to work day and night on the job in hand: it never has a day off. You become so used to your internal voice being part of your experience that, in the same way as a fish doesn't notice the water, you don't notice the voice. The difference is, of course the fish doesn't want to get out of the water, but you want and need the ability to be able to tune out the voice and recognize it is *in* your environment, but it is *not* your environment. It's so active because you have given it an impossible job to do. If you put the same workload on your physical body it simply would not cope. The sign of an overworked body is physical pain, the sign of an overworked psyche is fear and anxiety, as everyday it strives to come up with solutions to overcome the days 'problems' that are keeping you from all of your goals. It is constantly telling you to change something in your external environment in order to make things better, instead of controlling your internal environment.

The problem with this scenario is that many situations conflict. If you accept that the job of your unconscious mind is to keep you alive, safe, healthy, happy etc. and that your internal voice is simply commentating on the best options available at any given time, then what happens when you are presented with a heavy food that has made you fat, but that you love?

One of the ways you know your internal voice is simply a commentator or narrator and not the real 'you' is because it always gives you both options. Take this example, I will use cake but please insert any heavy food of your choice that you are regularly tempted by:

Voice 1: 'Ooh there's a cake – it looks soooooo good!'

Voice 2: *'You shouldn't have it, you know you need to lose weight.'*

Voice 1: 'Yes, I know, but it looks REALLY good.' (Pleasure centres activated.)

Voice 2: *'If you have it, you will regret it – you know you shouldn't.'*

Voice 1: 'Just one won't hurt – I'll start my diet tomorrow!'

You then eat cake.

Voice 2: *(Five minutes later) 'I should not have had that cake, I feel really bad now.'* (Associating the pain with being overweight that it *was not able to access at the time because the pleasure centres in the brain were firing).*

I have news – you do not have to do what your internal voice tells you to do! It's just a voice; it is not you. When you hear it say 'have the cake' you can take a second (slow thinking) and use the new associations you have made throughout this programme to present you with a different option so that you associate more pleasure with not having the cake than with having it. Think of the Peperami lady! When she said, 'It calls out to me!' she was creating the illusion that a vending machine speaks, when it was simply her internal voice. When I taught her to change the internal voice to, 'Eat me and I am going to ruin your wedding!' and gave it the sound of the Peperami in the advert, she didn't pay any attention to it. In fact, she laughed at it.

Exercise

Remember in the section on anchoring, one of the exercises was to hold a fattening food, look in the mirror and say to the food, 'You did this to me'. Let's take that one step further.

Think of a time when a food (or the sofa) calls out to you, or any other situation that contributes to being fat. Write down in the left column what your internal voice says that gets you to do the fat behaviour. If you are saying, 'I don't have an internal voice – I just do it!' That's your internal voice telling you, you don't have an internal voice. Take a moment and listen to what you say just before you do the fat thing.

Then close your eyes and image 'you' (you should be really familiar with this 'you' by now) in the future and go inside 'you' and listen to your future you's internal voice. It has a different script and probably different tone of voice, too. What is this internal voice saying that makes 'you' do something different?

In this version of the exercise, instead of just talking to the food, you are going to hear what you say to yourself to enrich your experience. Imagine 'you' being ridiculously happy and fire the positive anchor you created as you listen to your new voice. Run the movie several times so it becomes really familiar and comfortable. The emotion will activate your right hemisphere and the language and behaviour will be stored in your left hemisphere so that, together, they will be working to change your mind. This will automatically transform your body.

FAT VOICE	SLIM VOICE (TO THE FOOD)	SLIM VOICE TO SELF
Go on – you deserve it	You are not going to ruin my life	I am happy and in control

. . . .

The best way to change your internal voice is to first notice it, then notice that you have noticed it. Then change what it says and how it says it. If, sometimes, it runs the old dialogue, remember, it's just a voice. Like the Peperami voice, you don't have to do what it says; in fact, you can feel as empowered as that lady did by changing it.

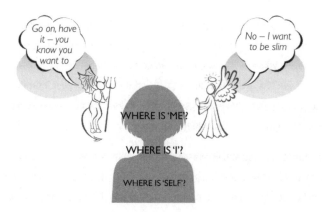

Recognize your S.H.I.T. thoughts and change them using CLEAN language.

Each time your internal voice runs negative dialogue reminding you of something that upset you that elicits a negative feeling, then you are reinforcing that neurological map. You are building negative associations and changing your 'brain juice' to produce more of the chemicals that make you feel bad.

When you run a negative commentary like this how long can you feel bad for? Minutes, hours, days? I have met people who have used the same commentary to feel bad for years! A negative thought produces enough brain chemicals to make you feel bad for just ninety seconds. If you feel bad for longer, it's because you keep repeating the thought. Each time you have it you ensure another ninety seconds of feeling bad. These ninety seconds soon add up! Changing your internal voice is an important way to address this, so whatever you are saying in your head that makes you feel bad, shut the **** up and say something else and you will only feel bad for the remainder of those ninety seconds. In the next chapter I will also teach you a couple of practical techniques to rapidly help collapse a negative feeling.

When we are talking about ourselves to ourselves, we often refer to 'us' in different tenses:

- 'I'
- 'Me'
- 'My Self'

Look at the following statement presented to me by a client when I asked her to write down what she wanted and why:

'I want to be slim, but there's a part of me that just keeps wanting to self-sabotage, even though I tell myself it's stupid I do it anyway. You know what it's like when you just can't stop yourself!'

It's easy to see the conflict: I, Me and Self are not all wanting the same thing. I wants to be slim and me keeps self-sabotaging. Finally, it's all blamed on 'you' who is an external representation.

In linguistics replacing the word 'you' with 'I' changes the meaning of the conversation and how it is processed internally. For example when a client says to me:

'I am so tired after work, I just stop at the takeaway. You know what it's like; you just can't resist; you can't help yourself.'

Just take a close look at that sentence and think about how the speaker is processing it internally. Her unconscious mind thinks she's talking about someone else so is not really associating any personal importance to the behaviour, or associating any pain with it. As soon as I got her to say:

'I am so tired after work, I just stop at the takeaway. I know what it's like; I just can't resist; I can't help myself.'

She looked strangely at me and said, 'That doesn't sound right. It makes me sound ridiculous; as if I have no control or no other choices!'

Just this one small change, always replacing 'you' with 'I', can be transformative, as it increases – you've guessed it – AWARENESS.

Exercise

In order to bring yourself harmony, complete the following sentences (you will find these in your journal as a permanent record, so do it there):

I want to lose weight because I will feel ....

Losing weight is the right thing for **me** as it will make **me** feel ....

Taking care of **myself** is important because I want to feel ....
of/with **myself**

Now look at the complete statement my client presented me with after this exercise:

> *'I have decided I am ready to be slimmer. Living life to the full and being healthy is really important to me now. I know I will be honouring and respecting myself by being healthy, and I know it will be so good for me in so many ways. Life will just be so much more fun! You know what it's like when you just know you've done the right thing? That's how I feel now.'*

When creating your new internal dialogue, bear in mind that talking in verbs (doing words) is better and more influential than using nouns (naming words). Look at these two examples:

I will be more disciplined (too general)

vs

I will consistently make better choices when I am ...(give a clear example of a situation)... (more specific)

I will use my willpower when faced with cakes (willpower is not a 'thing')

vs

I will remind myself of how it feels to feel good being slim every time I see a heavy cake (clear strategy easy to visualize)

. . . .

You are never not communicating with you – but you don't have to do what you hear. It's just a voice. You are the non-physical part of yourself that experiences life in a spiritual sense, which brings with it peace and tranquillity. Experienced meditators have learnt to quieten their voice so that they enjoy periods of silence that are blissful and peaceful. Meditation is one of the most effective ways to change your brain and numerous studies have shown that the benefits reach into all areas of your life. If you haven't already done so then I encourage to you go to a meditation class (most cities have a Buddhist centre which, far from promoting a religion, promotes a way of thinking that is quiet and harmonious) and they run cheap, or sometimes free, mediation classes. If you don't have a meditation class near you, there are some great books and online programmes that can help. The guided mediations in the Placebo Diet at Home programme will also strengthen your ability to find mind quiet.

Sometimes silence really is golden.

• •

Chapter 10

Tap In to Your Positivity

So far, you have learnt how your brain works, and some powerful techniques to change how you think and feel. Now I am going to show you an exciting and very simple therapy that you can use to eliminate, or 'collapse', negative feelings, such as cravings or lack of motivation. It's called Thought Field Therapy (TFT). My book, *Tapping For Life* (Hay House, 2009), explains more fully how this amazing technique works, and how it can be used specifically to collapse negative emotions, anxiety and past traumas, but this chapter offers a brief overview of the technique, specifically, how to stay positive and eliminate cravings.

People often overeat because of sadness, or some upset in an aspect of their lives. Dealing with these issues, so they stop affecting them on a day-to-day basis, is invaluable – not just for weight loss, but in order to move on in a positive way. When people come to see me for help with weight loss, I often begin by removing negative emotions, anxiety and even depression, and build self-esteem and self-worth before moving on to work on the issue of weight loss.

Earlier in the book we explored the fact that when people eat when they are not hungry, it's to get a *feeling*. Often, it's to get *any* feeling other than the one they are experiencing, and they seek solace in the sensation food gives them. They become *anchored* to feeling better when they eat. This is called 'comfort eating'. If you remove the causes of the negative feelings – whether it's a past trauma or anxiety, or a stress of some kind – the need to eat to get rid of that feeling by comfort eating disappears.

What then happens is that, as you start to feel better about yourself, you generally start to take more care of your body and you begin to lose weight without really trying. Changes that do need to be made become easier, because you know you really are worth the effort.

While I am going to give you an introduction to this amazing therapy and teach you some basic techniques, if you are suffering long-term effects of a past trauma or have ongoing anxiety then please go to www.powertochange.me.uk and download the free Stop Anxiety pack, which gives some TFT sequences and also includes a free MP3 guided meditation. If this is not sufficient, then I strongly encourage you to seek out a reputable therapist who can help you. Clearing emotional baggage is invaluable, not just for weight loss but for all areas of your life.

How Thought Field Therapy Works

Coming from an academic background, when I learnt how to use TFT I was keen to find out exactly how it works. In many ways some of the science behind it is still unconfirmed. What we do know is that it uses the meridian system, the invisible energy pathways used for centuries in traditional Chinese medicine, particularly in acupuncture. The Chinese identified the meridians as pathways that work like a circuit, flowing and conducting energy throughout the body. They believe that we store an imprint of our emotions within these pathways and that they are the link between the emotional mind and the body. It might be helpful to think of the meridians as 'emotional highways' or roads. If there's a crash on a road, it creates a blockage and traffic cannot flow. In the same way, a trauma or anxiety can cause a blockage in your meridians that prevents energy from flowing, causing emotional or physical distress, or both.

The developer of the technique of TFT, American psychologist Dr Roger Callahan, discovered that tapping on very specific points could clear these blockages. Whereas an acupuncturist would insert a needle, with TFT you simply 'tap' the same spot. You can do TFT on yourself – there are absolutely *no* harmful side effects and even if you do it wrong, it doesn't matter. It won't work, but you will do yourself absolutely no harm at all; it is the safest of all therapies. Gary Craig trained with Dr Callahan and went onto develop EFT (Emotional Freedom Technique). Ostensibly the main difference between the two tapping therapies is that with TFT you only tap on specific points, as Chinese medicine teaches us that each emotion has a prescription or algorithm that specifically targets that specific thought, whereas with EFT you tap all the points and repeat out loud statements or affirmations. Having trained with Dr Callahan myself, my own preference is for TFT, as it is more diagnostic and in my experience often works better, but of course that is not to say EFT doesn't work, it's a personal choice.

Measuring positive and negative

One of the most important concepts in TFT is that we can measure its effectiveness (apart from the fact that you can feel the emotion has gone or changed) using the polarity of your body. Every cell in your body has a polarity, it helps things get into and out of the cell with positive and negative ions. Your whole body also has a polarity, which can be tested using a standard electrician's voltmeter. When you are 'positive', cells can function normally and the process of growth and repair can take place naturally. When the cells' polarity is negative, however, healing and regeneration cannot take place. Imagine the battery in your TV remote being put in upside-down – the remote just won't work until you change it around to get the positive connection. Your body is the same. What is important is that negativity, as measured in terms of polarity, also affects us emotionally. When you are in a negative state all negative emotions are amplified – fears, cravings and all negative thoughts become more powerful and consuming.

In TFT this state is called 'Psychological Reversal' (PR), which is when your thoughts are the exact *opposite* of how you would like to feel – i.e. negative instead of positive. When you are 'reversed' you are prone to self-sabotage in your thoughts and your behaviours. Applied kinesiology uses a form of muscle testing to ascertain whether you are positive or negative when attuned to a certain thought. It's beyond the scope of this book (but explained in full in *Tapping For Life*) but, in simple terms, if you put your arm out to the side parallel with the floor and have someone gently press on your arm while you think of the person you love most in the world, or something you are really good at and love doing, you can easily resist this pressure and you're arm stays strong. However, if you think about someone you dislike or something you are really bad at, your arm will go weak and you will not be able to resist the pressure. This is another perfect example of how the mind and the body are totally connected and how a thought can affect you physiologically.

When you are 'reversed', this can be corrected by changing your state and your physiology – in other words your 'brain juice'. Physical exercise, and the generation of endorphins can correct the imbalance, but it's not always practical to put on some lively music and dance around laughing to generate an endorphin boost! Thankfully, TFT offers us a simpler way of restoring the correct balance – it's called the TFT Triangle. Through tapping on very specific meridian points that balance the body's energy, it can return us to 'positivity'.

Just like a battery has a positive and a negative charge at each end, your body also has both, and the palm of your hand is positive and the back of your hand negative. If you were to do the arm testing exercise described above, but instead of thinking a positive thought, have one arm outstretched, then bend the other arm and put the hand just above your head (not quite touching), palm facing downwards, the outstretched arm would test strong when pressed. However, if you were to turn the hand over your head so the palm faces upwards, the outstretched arm would test weak and you would not be able to resist the pressure. If this is what happens then that indicates you are in balance. However, if you test weak when the palm is facing the top of your head, you are in PR.

Imagine a cushion cover made of two different-coloured fabrics, one each side; there has to be a seam at the sides joining the two together. The side of your hand is the equivalent, it is not a seam but it is a meridian line, where the top of your hand meets the palm. It's the most important meridian point in the body for balancing polarity, so even just tapping the side of your hand when you feel a bit confused or flustered can be a very useful technique. Get in to the habit of doing this simple exercise regularly throughout the day, whenever you need a boost. If you are reversed, then it may correct it and if you are not, it won't do anything at all. It's totally harmless and yet, at the same time, can be immensely powerful. Many athletes are beginning to realize the power of maintaining a balance in order to perform at their best, especially when there's an intricate skill involved such as shooting or hitting a board accurately as in triple jump. I teach all my clients to do this before crucial meetings or when writing important articles.

Prevention is always better than cure so rather than waiting till you feel negative or start to self-sabotage, get into the habit of tapping the side of your hand every time you wash your hands.

For a stronger boost then the following sequence is very powerful.

Exercise: The TFT Triangle

If you have a negative thought, simply hold that thought and, using two or three fingers of one hand, tap on the following points firmly but not too hard for about 10 seconds each.

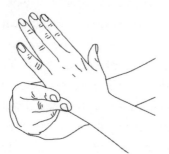

1. Side of hand

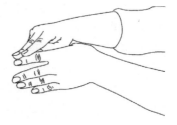

2. Index finger (if)

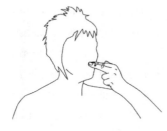

3. Under nose (un)

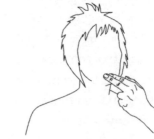

4. Under lip (ul)

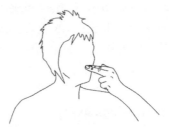

5. Repeat under nose (un)

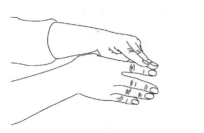

6. Index finger other hand (if)

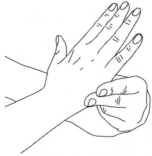

7. Side other hand (sh)

This sequence is called the 'triangle' because you start with one hand, work up to the face, and then work down to the other hand, making a triangle shape. Tapping can be used to remove any negative thought or feeling. You can use the 'triangle' to collapse negativity, but, as I have mentioned, it is also important to prevent negativity *before* it occurs, too, so get into the habit of doing the sequence every morning as you are doing your visualizations, and every evening before you go to sleep as you are doing your visualizations. This will ensure that the images are positive. I do the triangle every morning in the shower and every evening after I've cleaned my teeth. I also do it any time I get a negative or irrational thought, or when I just feel I need an emotional reboot.

• •

I taught you earlier how to use your mind to create a new neurological pathway to collapse the desire for a certain food. There is another TFT technique that also works well to collapse food cravings.

Exercise: Tapping Cravings Away

* Focus your mind on the food you crave – if possible, look at it and smell it so you are really 'in the thought'. Then rate the craving from 1–10, with 10 being a full-on craving and one being 'not bothered'.

* Tap the following points for approximately 10 seconds each:

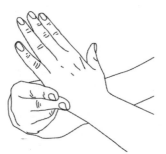

1. Side of hand

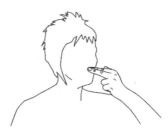

2. Under nose (un)

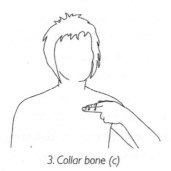

3. Collar bone (c)

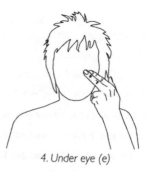

4. Under eye (e)

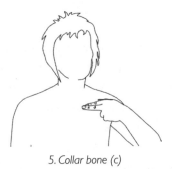

5. Collar bone (c)

- Then tap the gamut spot, on the back of your hand between the little finger and ring finger knuckles continually. As you do so, hum a few bars of a tune (e.g. 'Happy Birthday'), then count 1, 2, 3, 4, 5, out loud. Stop and then hum again.

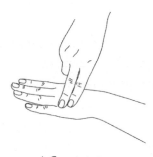

6. Gamut spot

- Still tapping, look down toward one shoulder, keeping your head still. Then look toward the other shoulder; then roll your eyes up and all the way round 360 degrees; then roll them around the other way.

- Tap the first sequence again.

- Now rate the craving on a scale of 1–10. It will probably have reduced. Repeat the entire process until the craving has gone. Then close your eyes and positively anchor the feeling of control you have established. Appreciate that you are not under the control of a craving, and that *you* get to choose what you put in, and as a result 'on', your body.

Exercise

Another technique that takes just a few seconds and can change your brain chemistry is to trace the infinity symbol on your forehead, across your third eye. You are highly sensitive to touch here and if you close your eyes, clear your mind and trace the symbol whilst taking two or three breaths it can genuinely change your 'brain juice'.

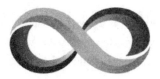

The infinity symbol

A good friend and colleague of mine, Kevin Laye, is working with neurologists to find out more about how this and other similar techniques can be used for rapid change. This exercise, along with the tapping of the side of your hand and the positive anchors we've already learned about, can all change and create new brain chemistry quickly.

Combining the techniques in the book with the colour-code nutrition system coming up, will give you all the tools you need to turn your life and your health around – for good.

PART II

How Your Body Works

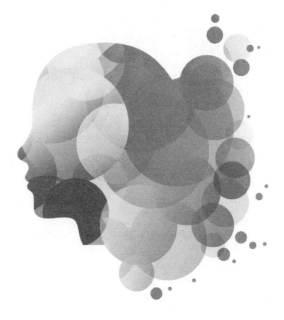

Chapter 11
Hormones R Us

So far in the book you have been learning how your brain works. In this part you will learn how your body works. When you combine the two things together you will have such a powerful sense of awareness that change will be inevitable *and* enjoyable.

The placebo effect also applies to food, although in this section there's nothing inert or 'fake' about the information you are being given, it's all based on sound nutrition advice and facts. If you know for sure what different foods do and how they make you feel, you don't need the placebo effect, but in the spirit of this book, let's look at what happens when you change how you think about a specific food.

Alia Crum, an Assistant Professor of Psychology at Stanford University, carried out a study demonstrating the placebo effect in operation when you think you are eating either a high- or low-calorie food.

- *Participants all drank the same 300-calorie, French vanilla shake, with one group believing they were drinking a 620-calorie, decadent 'Indulgence' shake and the other group thinking they were having a 140-calorie 'Sensishake' with a mere 140 calories and no fat or added sugar.*

- *Those who were given the 'Indulgence' labelled shake reported greater satiety (they felt fuller), but the bigger news was to come.*

- *While the 'Sensishake' group showed relatively stable ghrelin response (a key hunger-stimulating hormone), the 'Indulgence' group demonstrated a dramatic drop in ghrelin – about three times greater than those who thought they were drinking a low-calorie shake. Those in the indulgence group physically responded as if they had consumed excess calories.*

This clearly shows that how you think about food changes your physiology. By this point in the book that should not surprise you at all!

For many years the process of weight loss has been simplified into the phrase, 'Eat less – move more'. This is true – for most people, however it ignores the fact that we are all dependent on our body's physiology and there are a few variables that make it easier for some people to lose weight than others. It is important to understand that all your body's systems, including fat storing and fat burning, can be trained to be more or less efficient. Much of this is down to your nutrition and your lifestyle choices.

The good news is that, with the rare exception of some individuals with serious, diagnosed medical conditions, the way that your body stores and burns fat can be completely changed and retrained. The medical conditions that do adversely affect metabolism present early in life, so any medical diagnosis will have been identified during adolescence at the latest and will have other accompanying symptoms as well as weight gain. In other words, you cannot use your genes as an excuse.

*Don't blame it on your genes when
you can't get into your jeans.*

To help you absorb the information and start to think about how you can put it into practice (which as you know means creating new neurological maps to make it automatic), there are some short exercises that you can complete in your journal to help ignite the fuse for the changes you want to make. When you have finished this book, you will certainly benefit from dipping into and out of it and rereading certain sections to remind you of all you have learnt. Your journal, however, is a working document that is personal to you. Research has shown over and over again that people who keep journals when they want to change something, massively increase their chances of making permanent change. Keep it somewhere you can dip in and out of it to remind yourself of some of the practical exercises you have already and which you should keep going back to.

Step-by-step Weight Loss

1. Change Your Mind (Brain)

2. Manage Your Hormones and Your Metabolism

3. Result = Transform Your Body

In this and the next chapter you are going to learn how your body can be turned from a highly efficient, fat-storing machine into a highly efficient fat-burning machine, simply by making some key changes to the balance of your diet (and without having to spend hours at the gym!). An unhealthy body is great at storing fat, but rubbish at burning it. A healthy body, on the other hand, is great at burning fat and rubbish at storing it. The good news is – you get to choose which way your body works.

The different systems in the body are interconnected and their combined effects give us optimum health. When it comes to weight loss, the most important systems, or factors, are those shown in the graphic below.

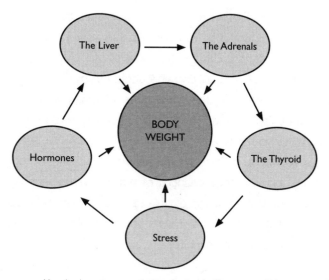

Your body systems work together and affect your weight

The Liver

Let's start with the liver, because it's arguably the most important organ when it comes to weight loss. When you think of your digestive system, you probably think of your stomach, your intestines and your bowels, but you probably don't think about your liver. Yet this key organ is not only responsible for filtering everything that goes through your body (just like an oil filter on a car), it also has a huge impact on how you metabolize and store food as energy – and how you make that energy available for use, as and when needed.

Although the liver is an organ, it is also considered a gland, because it produces bile. A poorly functioning liver can cause fluid to leak into the area just below the rib cage, giving a potbelly appearance. Unlike rolls of fat, this sac of fluid feels more solid and can actually be pushed from side to side. A dysfunctional liver is caused by a lack of nutrients and an imbalanced diet. Your liver will produce obvious physical symptoms if it is not looked after. As well as the potbelly, you may notice that your tongue looks white and furry and has a crease down the centre. You may have severe, on-going itching, pain in the right shoulder, liver spots, or a yellow colour to the skin or the whites of the eyes known as jaundice. People with a poorly functioning liver often suffer from bloating, especially after eating gluten, which is found in grains. Rice and corn are safe for coeliac patients (who cannot tolerate even minute amounts of gluten), but wheat, barley and rye are not.

More serious liver conditions include hepatitis – inflammation of the liver – and cirrhosis – a late stage of liver disease that causes a build-up of scar tissue. Although a dysfunctional liver can inhibit fat burning, and therefore weight loss, a severely dysfunctional and diseased liver usually results in drastic weight loss.

Despite all the symptoms of physical stress, an overworked liver retains an amazing capacity to perform its functions, which explains why so many people have advanced liver dysfunction before being diagnosed. If you think you may have the symptoms of a severely dysfunctional liver, go to www.britishlivertrust.org.uk for more information. If you are still concerned, consult your GP. If you think you may have some signs of a slightly dysfunctional liver, which may be contributing to your weight gain, then this chapter and the colour coded nutrition system in Chapter 14 will show you how you can help correct it naturally.

What the Liver Does

The liver is situated on the right-hand side, at the bottom of the rib cage, and it is directly 'plumbed into' the digestive system and the heart for circulation. It has many functions, including the following:

- Production of bile – required for the digestion of fats

- Filtering of hormones

- Converting the extra glucose in the body into stored glycogen in liver cells; and then converting it back into glucose for energy when needed

- Production of blood-clotting factors

- Production of amino acids (the building blocks for making proteins), including those used to help fight infection

- Processing and storage of iron – essential for red blood cell production

- Manufacture of cholesterol for growth and repair, and other chemicals required for fat transport

- Conversion of waste products of body metabolism into urea, which is then excreted in the urine

- Metabolization of medications into their active ingredients in the body.

A healthy liver is essential for effective, long-term weight loss but it can be stressed or damaged by several factors. Here are some of the key ones:

- Alcohol

- A high intake of sugar

- A diet low in nutrients

- A diet high in caffeine

- Long-term use of certain medications
- Smoking.

HELP WITH STOPPING SMOKING

If you are a smoker and would like to stop – please go to www. powertochange.me.uk and download my free Stop Smoking pack. It includes some tapping exercises plus a guided mediation. Listen to this for a few nights just before you go to sleep. I don't charge for this pack, as even the thought that it might save or extend one life is more than enough pay back for me. If it works for you (the success rate is very high) please get any other smokers you know to do the same and have it with my compliments.

If you are serious about wanting to lose weight, for the next few weeks spend some time looking after your liver and the whole process of burning fat will become much easier. I will tell you specifically how to do this, of course! And not only in this chapter – the colour-code system has been designed to promote healthy liver function.

Here are some foods that promote a healthy liver:

- **Cruciferous vegetables**, for example, broccoli, cauliflower, Brussels sprouts, kale, cabbage, pak choi. These all contain vitamins, minerals and fibre. As well as aiding digestion and fat burning, they contain phytochemicals that can stimulate enzymes in the body that detoxify carcinogens before they damage cells, helping prevent cancer.
- **Foods containing sulphur**, such as garlic, legumes, onions and eggs.
- **Good sources of water-soluble fibre**, including pears, oat bran, apples and legumes.

- **Artichokes, beets, carrots, dandelion, cranberries (and most other berries), turmeric and cinnamon.**
- **Good-quality protein foods**, such as fish, tofu or organic chicken.

As the liver is a detoxifying organ, it's important to maintain good levels of hydration to flush toxins out once the liver has processed them.

Constipation can cause liver problems because the bowel isn't able to excrete the toxins through the faeces, so they stay in the body and have to be cleared by the liver. Therefore a diet high in fibre is indirectly linked to the health of the liver.

It can take years of abuse to severely impair liver function, but once the damage is done, a good, detoxifying diet and a reduction in stress can rejuvenate this organ, often in just a few months. You are likely to notice a difference in energy levels and improved digestion after just two weeks of eating a vegetable-rich diet that also contains high-quality proteins such as fish and organic chicken. The colour-code system makes this really easy to achieve.

Exercise

Based on what you have just read, think of three things that you can start doing *now* that will boost your liver function, and therefore your ability to burn fat. Now write them down – this is important, because it makes you focus, and it uses a different part of your brain than just thinking it. So just do it! When you have written the three things down, say them out loud to make a statement (you know from earlier chapters how powerful this is). You can use the exercise in your journal if you find it easier than writing in the book. As you do this, visualize these changes *actually happening* inside your body. Let's say for example that you write for the first one:

I will make a cranberry and mixed-berry fruit smoothie every day, or, **I will eat more green-coloured vegetables.** You then say exactly that out loud and add at the end, 'And it will help me become healthy and slim'. You have to mean this as you say it, and of course, you know you must attach emotion to it. Each morning, as you drink your smoothie, say the words and then visualize how healthy the smoothie is making you as you drink it. In this way you create positive anchors to it, and you change your mental and your physical physiology at the same time. The ultimate winning combination!

Do this for each of your three liver-boosting ideas:

1. ....

2. ....

3. ....

Hormones as Chemical Messengers

The collective term for all the glands that produce and secrete hormones is the 'endocrine system'. Hormones are chemical messengers created by the body; they transfer information from one set of cells to another to coordinate the functions of different parts of the body. Hormones regulate the body's growth and metabolism (all the physical and chemical processes of the body), as well as sexual development and function. Hormones are released into the bloodstream and may affect one or several organs throughout the body. In the case of weight loss, if even one hormone is out of balance, then others can be affected, restricting your body's ability to burn fat.

Once hormones have been produced by glands, they are released into the bloodstream as needed; they are a bit like letters or parcels that have been written and are waiting to be posted. These parcels are being sent all over your body 24/7, and determine your metabolic rate and to a large extent how your body functions.

Each hormone has a specific role. For example, insulin lowers blood sugar and converts excess glucose into fat, while glucagon increases blood sugar and promotes fat burning to provide energy in between meals. For a constant supply of energy without the highs and lows, these two hormones must work in balance. We will look at the vital role insulin plays in weight loss in more detail a little later on.

Just as a parcel can be sent recorded delivery, each hormonal message sent to a cell demands a receipt or a response. The cells have receivers, much like a letterbox, through which they receive the information. If the receiver is blocked it's like a letterbox being the wrong shape and the parcel cannot be delivered. There are times when you are producing the right hormone, but it is being blocked from doing its work. This is called a 'feedback system' and in this way information passes between the glands and the brain to decide how much of a particular hormone is needed; in a healthy body, production and release of all hormones is balanced.

Oestrogen

An example of when this system doesn't work is when chemicals that mimic hormones – such as pesticides – enter the bloodstream, or when hormones in the food chain are consumed, throwing our own hormone production out of balance by disrupting the feedback mechanism. One example of this is oestrogen. This is a female sex hormone that is involved in reproduction and also in fat storage. It is oestrogen that directs fat to be stored just under the belly button and on the hips and thighs; after menopause, when these levels drop, fat deposition changes and you often see older women with lovely slim legs and big round tummies. If you have elevated oestrogen levels, then you are in fat-storing mode (fat cells themselves produce oestrogen).

As well as your naturally produced oestrogen, you may be consuming oestrogen in your diet if you eat a lot of farmed meat because the hormone is often used in animal feed. Chickens fed on a diet high in growth hormones can grow rapidly and be big enough to slaughter in six weeks, instead of the 22 weeks it would take them to grow and develop naturally. Animal feeds that contain a cocktail of hormones to promote rapid growth are highly lucrative and widely used. It is no coincidence that, since hormones have started indirectly entering our food chain in this way, and the contraceptive pill has increased the amount of oestrogen in the water, the age of puberty has reduced. Men are also having more problems with fertility – and some even develop 'man boobs'.

Hormones not only control your appetite, the drive to eat and where fat is stored, but as you know from your own experience, they also affect your mood. We have already looked at the ability of serotonin to make us feel relaxed, less stressed and less prone to cravings. There's another hormone that makes us feel good. It's called oxytocin, and it's produced in the hypothalamus.

Oxytocin

Oxytocin is a really important hormone that also functions as a neurotransmitter. (These are the ferry-like molecules that transport signals across the synapse to carry information through the brain and create new maps). Oxytocin is often called the 'cuddle hormone' and Cupid's arrow is said to have been dipped in it! We release oxytocin when we feel love, trust and comfort, and it can be even more powerful than serotonin. If you need a lift, you can tap into the power of simply spending time with your family and friends and, of course, your loved one. Even interacting with pets can release hormones that make us feel good; several studies have shown the therapeutic benefits of dog 'visitors' to long-term patients in hospitals and homes. When you are happy, contented and not under stress, the drive to eat when you're not hungry disappears.

Someone who knows more than most about the effects of oxytocin and the placebo effect is David Hamilton. A former research scientist involved in many drug trials, he witnessed first-hand just how many people spontaneously heal due to the placebo effect. I recommend reading David's great book, *Why Kindness Is Good for You*, for more detailed information on how and why we feel good.

Let's go back to the example of the McVitie's digestive biscuit advert described earlier (if you are following the online programme, you will have seen the advert, too). Do you remember, the biscuit was portrayed as a kitten coming out of a packet? When I show this advert in my workshops and seminars you can hear the 'oooohs' and 'ahhhhs' as the kitten pokes its cute head out of the packet. In this instant when you have this response, oxytocin is being produced.

It's such a powerful neurotransmitter that it can affect many neurons simultaneously, a bit like a chemical solution flowing through your brain, making it easy for new neurological pathways to be created. In other words, it's easier to permanently change your mind when your brain is full of oxytocin. The theory, which is impossible to prove but makes perfect sense, comes from the fact that men and women are different (no surprises there), which means when they meet and form a relationship, in order to ensure procreation of the species they have to get on, at least for long enough to have sex enough times to reproduce! That means they have to change how they think and feel about certain things in order to accommodate the other persons needs. Have you even known someone who hated doing something, and then got in a new relationship and then suddenly embraced this thing or behaviour? Seemingly quite happily! This is because of the effects of oxytocin.

Let's link back to the anchoring exercise to see its relevance here. When you can elicit a genuine feeling of happiness by firing an anchor, you are creating the perfect environment inside your brain for change – and the creation of new behaviours. So the more positive thoughts, dialogue and, most importantly, feelings that you can generate when eating new lighter foods, the more new neurological pathways you create that will make you slim. Simple isn't it! You just have to learn how to feel good.

Insulin

Insulin is one of the better-known hormones, and like all hormones, it is essential for health. Simply put, one of insulin's main functions in the body is to control what goes into and out of cells, including glucose and fat. Insulin is largely responsible for maintaining optimal blood glucose levels, as a rise *or* a fall in blood glucose can have serious consequences for our health.

Glucose is the primary energy source in our bodies and *every* cell needs it. It makes sense therefore that we have the right amount circulating in our blood so it can be delivered to our cells. It is insulin's job to monitor and maintain blood glucose levels and respond to changing requirements. Clearly, the demand for fuel goes up when we are active, but glucose alone can't meet all our needs for energy because we just don't store enough of it (an average adult stores just over 2,000 calories as glucose). So when levels get low, we add fat to the mixture (we can store literally billions of calories of this) to make up the deficit.

Think of a hybrid car. It is designed to run on two fuels – electricity (via a battery) and petrol (or diesel) from the storage tank. The amount of charge in the battery, and the power required by the engine at any given time, determine which fuel is used. When battery levels are fully charged and energy demand is low – for example when we are pottering around at low speed – no petrol is needed because the battery can meet all the demands for energy. However, on longer distances and at a higher speed, the battery charge drops quickly, so the car burns petrol as well as using the charge from the battery to make up the deficit.

In much the same way, the amount of glucose in your blood determines how much fat you burn in relation to the demands for energy. When glucose levels are high, and activity is low to moderate, little fat is needed, but when glucose levels are low and energy requirements go up, you need to add fat to the mixture to keep the supply constant. For effective fat burning and weight loss, then, you need a combination of glucose *and* fat (as you will see in Chapter 12, which looks at exercise). While you can burn glucose without fat, *you cannot burn fat without glucose.*

If there's too much circulating glucose, you use this for energy instead of burning fat to bring blood glucose levels down naturally; insulin makes sure of this by blocking fat burning, and any excess glucose that can't be burned as fuel is converted into fat. This process is initiated by insulin, so you can see what a vital role this hormone plays in weight loss.

Insulin Resistance

In a healthy person, the pancreas produces insulin. In someone with type 1 diabetes, the pancreas cannot produce it, so it has to be injected. Years ago, people with this type of diabetes simply deteriorated and died. Today it is a manageable condition rather than a disease. In type 2 diabetes the body does produce insulin but it is not usable – the cells cannot respond to it as they should. Medication is used to correct this, and diet and exercise also play a key role. In many cases type 2 diabetes is reversible with a good regime.

In recent years a new condition that is also characterized by the body's inability to use insulin has been discovered. Similar in part to type 2 diabetes, it is called insulin resistance, or IR. The condition is also the cause of polycystic ovary syndrome, or PCOS (an imbalance of hormones that can cause serious health problems and infertility), because hyperinsulinemia (high insulin) has an impact on ovarian function. There is also a strong link between insulin and the adrenals (as you will see, many of the symptoms of imbalance are similar), as the whole endocrine system has to be in balance for optimum health.

The reality is that most people who are obese are probably insulin resistant. If you think about the word 'resistant', it gives you a clue as to what the condition actually means. Something is preventing something else from happening. Have you ever tried to unlock a door with a key that seems to fit into the lock, yet the mechanics aren't quite right and the key won't turn? That's exactly what happens with insulin resistance: the lock on the cell doesn't recognize insulin as the key and prevents it from working.

Remember the description earlier about the parcel being sent recorded delivery? Imagine it can't be delivered now because there's no one there to sign for it. When this happens in IR, blood sugar levels don't go down (as insulin is struggling to get it into cells), so the body produces more and more insulin to try and get the job done. It's a bit like shouting if someone can't hear you – if they are deaf, it doesn't matter how loud you shout, they won't hear. As a result of this increase in insulin production, fat burning is blocked.

Here are some of the non-medical symptoms of insulin resistance:

- Feeling tired even after a full night's sleep
- Inability to get to sleep, or waking in the early hours
- Giddiness when moving from a seated position to standing
- Stretch marks and brown pigments in the skin
- Unexplained fatigue
- Weight gain – especially in the mid-section
- Erratic or painful periods
- Inability to focus or concentrate
- Intestinal bloating and gas
- Tired after eating
- Difficulty losing weight
- Facial hair, or any excessive hair (in women)
- Mood swings
- Depression
- Excessive hunger and food cravings.

Medical symptoms include:

- High circulating insulin levels
- High blood glucose

- Increased blood triglycerides (fats)
- Increased blood pressure.

Although insulin resistance is a relatively 'new' condition, the association between a disorder of carbohydrate metabolism (balancing blood sugar) and the endocrine system (glands and hormones) was first described as early as 1921. Even today, many GPs are only just being informed of the significance of this condition, and as a result many people have to seek a private diagnosis because traditional glucose tolerance tests can't diagnose insulin resistance and the IR test is not available through many GPs. For more information on how to get tested privately visit www.medichecks.com. They will send a nurse out to collect your blood and give you a professional analysis and report, as well as a telephone consultation when your results are ready.

Even if you are IR, the nutrition guidelines will be exactly the same as I'm giving you in this programme. This will become much clearer when you have read the exercise and nutrition sections *(see chapters 12 and 13)* and have seen the simplicity of the colour-code system. In addition to what you eat, *you must exercise* in order to change your hormonal production and balance. Sitting around and being inactive is a cause of fatness, not a cure. If you are IR and you do not address it, you are at increased risk of heart disease and other conditions, not just diabetes.

In a normal, healthy body the natural production of insulin works very well on a simple 'feedback system' (messages being sent recorded delivery and being signed for): we eat, blood sugar goes up, and the right amount of insulin is released to put the glucose into the cells that need it. While glucose levels are high, insulin stops fat from being used for energy, as it's simply not needed. When the circulating glucose levels drop, and energy requirements are not being met, then fat is released to make up the difference.

An insulin resistant body may have an insulin response 5–10 times greater than a healthy body, which means you go into fat storing mode five times earlier. This explains why some people can eat the same foods as others and not gain fat. Some of this may be genetic, but these genes can be 'turned off' and hormones up-regulated or down-regulated depending on your lifestyle. So, the good news is, with the right nutrition, and regular exercise to improve your body's composition and reduce the ratio of fat to muscle (lean body mass – or LBM), you can restore the balance. It won't happen overnight though – it will take time to get your body into the healthy state you desire and become a fat burner.

Make it a priority to manage your blood sugar, because it is high blood sugar (or glucose) that triggers the extra insulin release and the subsequent increase in fat storing. If you focus on preventing high blood glucose, rather than losing weight at any cost, the fat and the inches will come off automatically. You will also feel so much better!

A Personal Story about Insulin Resistance

I was lucky enough to meet Professor Nadir Rashad Farid, a brilliant endocrinologist whose pioneering work on insulin resistance (IR) helped my daughter Emilie get the diagnosis she needed after several years of feeling unwell, suffering some of the extremely unpleasant symptoms of IR and PCOS, and struggling with her weight. When Emilie was 16 (she's now 25), we were told that everything she was going through was normal for her age but I knew this was not the case, and I was determined to find a way to help her.

I knew in my heart, and through my training, that nutrition and exercise were key, but I didn't know exactly what the problem was. After watching Professor Farid speak at a seminar, I immediately recognized the symptoms of IR in Emilie. I just sat and cried, partly with relief because I'd finally found some answers, and partly with concern for her future.

I spoke to Professor Farid after the seminar and he immediately agreed to see Emilie. Thanks to him, she now has a clear strategy to manage her condition and some serious health consequences have been avoided before they fully began. With a type I diabetic grandmother (insulin dependent), Emilie was genetically predisposed to problems, but now, with the right nutrition and exercise, she is likely to avoid becoming diabetic. I have no doubt that she would now be in a very different place, health-wise, if I hadn't attended the seminar that day. This experience also allowed me to share this vital information from one of the world's leading experts with you now. Sadly Professor Farid has passed away, but he leaves an amazing legacy.

More About Glucose

You may have heard athletes use the term 'hitting the wall'. This refers to the point in extreme exercise when there is no more glucose left in the body. We have a 'survival mechanism' to deal with this – it's a special facility that is designed to protect us in times of famine. However, as you will see, when we diet it's easy to trick the body into using this mechanism. When blood glucose is getting low, we use more and more fat mixed with the glucose to make it last longer; you could say fat dilutes the glucose to keep the energy supply going, but eventually, with extreme exercise such as marathon running, glucose runs out.

When this happens we literally cannibalize our own muscle tissue to release the tiny glucose strands within the muscle to provide us (primarily our brains) with the energy we need to function. This state is called 'ketosis'. This was a very useful mechanism for our hunter-gatherer ancestors, who had times of famine and had to go hunting all day to chase and catch their food. Today, ketosis can be initiated in exactly the same way, simply by eating a high-protein, low-carb diet.

You will learn more about this in later chapters, but just think about that and let me repeat it again because it is hugely important:

When we run out of glucose, we cannibalize our muscle tissue (lean body mass, or LBM) to provide the brain with the glucose it needs. This is significant because the only place in our body that burns fat is muscle (LBM). When you cannibalize LBM, you are reducing your ability to burn fat.

In my view, Dr Atkins had it half right when he 'created' his high-protein diet, but sadly his approach (and those of the others who jumped on the same lucrative bandwagon) failed to appreciate the overall consequence on body composition, and overall health. His principle was simple: if insulin causes fat storage and blocks fat burning, then let's create a system to prevent insulin from being produced. Then we can't get fat! Sounds too good to be true, eh? It is. We *need* insulin, and when we deliberately suppress insulin production it triggers a series of chain reactions that lead to long-term health problems, some of which can be fatal. This is why we give diabetics insulin – without it we die!

The ketones (produced when we are in ketosis) are a by-product of fat metabolism and are used for energy when circulating glucose is dangerously low. Your brain (which has a dominant need for glucose) does not function well on ketones and it is certainly *not* a desirable condition. So much of our behaviour, including cravings and the ability to stay motivated, depends on our brain getting exactly the right amount of glucose, so it's common sense to avoid 'running it' on substandard fuel. That's what you are effectively doing if you are in ketosis. If you want a healthy body, you first have to have a healthy brain.

If your GP tests your urine and detects ketones, you have been officially diagnosed with a metabolic dysfunction. Yet for some reason in the high-protein community, this dysfunction is seen as a success – even desirable! You are told to go to the chemist to buy a kit to measure your own urine so you can make sure you *are* in ketosis! Glucose in the right amount, is brain food; you must have it.

Millions of people, all chasing the promise of weight loss, flocked like lemmings to follow this advice. That's very scary! I have no doubt that Dr Atkins was well intentioned, but the potential long-term effects of a high-protein diet include kidney failure, heart disease and osteoporosis, to name but a few. Several deaths have been attributed to this regime, too – well, that's certainly one way to lose weight! The answer is to manage our insulin levels so we produce enough to maintain normal healthy function, but avoid the overproduction, or 'spiking', caused by eating foods that contain too much glucose.

This is one of the key components in the colour-code system – you eat foods that release their glucose slowly, so you don't get the insulin 'spikes' that cause weight gain. You will see when you follow the colour code guidelines how simple this can be. This chapter is just to give you an understanding of how and why the colour-code system works so well. My own studies have shown that when you understand the principles behind any system you are following, and you have confidence in it, it's easier for your unconscious mind to accept all the new things you are learning, and you can easily adapt your behaviours to make the changes you need to make.

So, now you understand how balancing your hormones is crucial for weight loss – both physiologically and emotionally. Let's now have a look at some specific glands and how you can boost your fat-burning potential naturally.

The Adrenals

The adrenal glands sit at the top of the kidneys and are largely responsible for managing your body's stress levels. When you are under stress, you produce a different set of hormones than you do when you are relaxed and peaceful. Because your energy requirements are different when you are stressed, this directly affects fat storage. When your adrenals are stressed, you store more fat – typically around the mid-section – you may also notice some facial hair, a bloated face and puffy eyes.

Your adrenals control your sleep patterns via circadian rhythms so when they are stressed you don't achieve peaceful, restful sleep and find you are tired all day. Despite being 'exhausted' by the time you go to bed, you can't sleep, or you wake up at 2 a.m. for no apparent reason and can't get back to sleep for ages. You may also notice that you get out of breath easily and are more prone to stress – little things make you anxious, you develop a very short fuse and worry a lot. You may get very thirsty but despite consuming lots of fluids, the reduced sodium levels associated with this condition make it difficult for water to be absorbed into the cells, so you remain dehydrated. Some of the body's serotonin is produced by the adrenals and as you now know, this can lead to an increase in cravings.

Here are some guidelines for keeping your adrenals healthy.

- Avoid high-sugar foods.
- Avoid refined foods, even if they contain no visible added sugar.
- Eat slow-releasing foods (as listed at the top of the arrows – *pages 239 and 244*).
- Avoid too much caffeine.
- Avoid getting really hungry.
- Eat healthy, good-quality snacks, such as fruit and nuts.
- Eat high-quality proteins like fish (wild or organic); organic chicken; organic beans and lentils; lean, lightly cooked red meat (rare meat is easier to digest); and fresh, raw nuts.
- Eat lots of raw and lightly cooked vegetables (including salads).
- Avoid artificial sweeteners.
- Reduce stress levels.

The Thyroid

This is the gland that regulates your body's metabolism. In other words, it controls the speed at which you burn fuel. Many years ago it was thought of as a totally superfluous organ as no one really knew what it did, but today we have a much better understanding of its importance.

The thyroid works a bit like the accelerator in a car – you can either go faster or slower depending on the environment. If you go faster, you burn more fuel; if you go slower you conserve fuel.

The environment in this case is determined by your hormones – how much (and what) you are eating, how active you are and your overall health. The thyroid also determines your body temperature, just like a thermostat.

The thyroid is situated in the throat and, if it is dysfunctional, can appear quite large. An overactive thyroid means your metabolic rate is too high. Extreme weight loss occurs, you become irrational, and your eye sockets can contract, giving the appearance of protruding eyeballs. An underactive thyroid means the reverse – sufferers become sluggish, mentally and physically fatigued, and gain weight that is difficult to shift. This weight tends to be general and not as site-specific as when your liver is dysfunctional (potbelly) or your adrenals are stressed (tummy).

There is a strong link between your thyroid gland and your ovaries, which produce oestrogen. This is especially relevant after menopause, a time when a lot of women gain weight. The majority of thyroid function occurs through the liver, where thyroid hormones are broken down, so a healthy liver is vital. Exercise can also stimulate thyroid function, and there's more about this a little later in the book.

To boost thyroid function you need to combine regular exercise with a nutrient-rich diet. Iodine is the key nutrient required for thyroid function and a deficiency in it will lead to an underactive thyroid.

Here are some foods that are rich in iodine:

- Sea vegetables (i.e. kelp)
- Yoghurt
- Cow's milk (stick to organic if possible)
- Eggs (preferably organic)
- Strawberries

- Mozzarella cheese
- Fish and shellfish.

Exercise

Think about and then list three things you can do every day that will increase your thyroid function and therefore your ability to burn fat. Then read them out loud, as you did for the previous exercises, and make a note in your journal.

1. ....

2. ....

3. ....

Stress

De-stressing is an undervalued component of weight loss. I've had clients take up yoga and think that it must somehow be burning more calories than aerobics because they start to lose weight despite having been previously 'stuck'! The reality is this: when you are stressed you release cortisol, which blocks the fat-burning process. If you blast away like a bat out of hell on the treadmill after a hard day at the office you put your body under a different kind of stress. Even if you enjoy it, it's still a form of stress and can reduce the amount of fat you can burn after exercise.

I'm not suggesting that you shouldn't do aerobic exercise – far from it. You *should* do aerobic exercise and resistance training to maximize fat burning! But you must also find a way of exercising, or some other technique, such as meditation, that relaxes you and doesn't over-stress your body. It may be that you do the aerobics class, but then finish with some yoga or meditation to relax and balance your hormones.

Believe me, when you do this you'll not only burn more fat after your exercise, you'll sleep better and your body will be able to complete the valuable process of growth and repair undisturbed by stress hormones. Learning to meditate, and doing it for just 10 minutes before you go to sleep, can be a great way to de-stress and balance your hormones for the body's nighttime processes. Your body produces some of the growth hormones responsible for fat burning at night, when you are in restful sleep. If you don't achieve restful sleep, you produce very few of these hormones and long-term fat metabolism is impaired.

Exercise

Think about and then write down three things you can do every day that will reduce your stress levels and therefore increase your ability to burn fat. You could try some of the psychological exercises from earlier in the book. Use the technique of repeating them out loud described earlier. Do it – it's important. If you are too lazy to do this, then why are you reading this book!? Just do it!

1. ....

2. ....

3. ....

Feeding Your Mind

Like all other body systems, your brain function is entirely dependent on receiving the right nutrients. Your brain weighs about 1.3kg (3lbs). Excluding water, 60% of the brain is made from fat.

You learned earlier that neurons (made from amino acids) are the functional units of the brain that send and receive messages about your internal and external environment. They also control your mood and how you feel generally. As everything we do is to get a feeling, then feeding our brain the right nutrients to do its job at an optimum level makes sense. A neurotransmitter carries a signal through the dendrites across the synapse to receptors in the next neuron, when the electrical signal (message) is received; this neuron acts on the message.

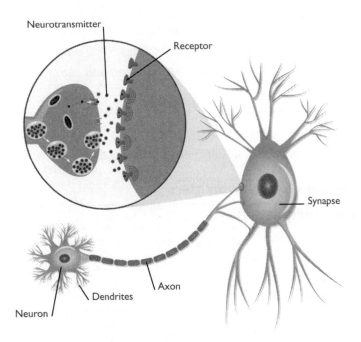

Information passes from one neuron to another through the synapse.

Collectively, neurotransmitters (NTs) such as dopamine and serotonin send messages to receptors, which control how we feel and what we do. Cravings and addictions occur when this delicate and precise process is out of balance.

When we produce more dopamine, which is a 'good feeling' NT, we feel much more motivated and alert. But after a while the receptors shut down so that 'normal' levels can be regained. It might sound like we are spoiling our own fun, however in terms of survival it makes sense. If we were in a constant state of bliss then we would be less likely to be processing new, potentially dangerous information or situations. Any high or low is, after a while, naturally reset to a mid-range level.

Most of the actions and behaviours we choose are reward based: when we have optimal (not too much and not too little) amounts of the right NTs, we feel balanced and can adapt to ever-changing situations.

We eat because that gives us a good feeling. We eat certain foods because they give us a better feeling than others. Generally chocolate produces a better reward than cabbage!

Feel-good Neurotransmitters

NEUROTRANSMITTER	FEELING	FOUND IN
Dopamine, adrenaline, noradrenaline	Higher energy, in control, motivated	Seaweed, spirulina, soy protein, eggs, cottage cheese, oily fish, turkey
Endorphins and enkephalins	Bliss, euphoric, reduce pain	Beef, turkey, liver, chicken; fish: cod, crab, lobsters, mussels, oysters, tuna, salmon, sardines
Serotonin	Mellow, confident, stable, connected	Turkey, beef, tuna, halibut, salmon, sardines, cod and scallops
GABA (gamma-aminobutyric acid) metabolic by-product of plants and microorganisms	Chilled, reduces anxiety and is calming	While GABA is not found in fresh food, it can be found in fermented foods, and certain foods can stimulate your body to produce more of it.**

** Flavonoids are phytonutrients found in plant-based foods, tea and wine and are known to have powerful antioxidant, anti-cancer and heart-protective properties. Flavonoids may also enhance GABA function.

Neurotransmitters are manufactured from amino acids (proteins) and are specific shapes that each fit into a specific receptor, just like a child's toy where the correct shapes have to be fitted in the correct hole. Unfortunately, many ingestible stimulants can mimic these shapes and interfere with the process. Once the receptor has been activated (no matter what by) it responds accordingly.

Eating the right amino acids is the first part of a two-part process. You also have to be able to convert them into NTs and this process is disrupted by alcohol, nicotine and caffeine. It is dependent on B vitamins, zinc and magnesium.

Addictions originate in the limbic system where our pleasure centres form part of our survival instinct. When we associate something pleasurable with survival, our limbic system automatically creates a compulsion for it. However, it cannot differentiate between naturally pleasurable substances and harmful or artificial substances. If you are ingesting something that instigates the exact same chemical reactions as dopamine, serotonin or endorphins, then these unnatural substances take over their role and we crave them. This is because we instinctively crave anything that makes us feel good, even if it's unhealthy and physically not good for us at all. Examples include:

- Cocaine docks into the same receptor sites as dopamine.
- Caffeine docks into the same receptor sites as dopamine.
- Heroin docks into the same receptor sites as endorphins.
- Alcohol docks into the same receptor sites as GABA.

When we have our first coffee of the day, we get a 'hit' that makes us feel good. If caffeine intake increases over time, we become desensitized to it, as receptors shut down; just like a thermostat self-monitors and is always looking to maintain homeostasis, neither too hot nor too cold.

If you continue to consume a stimulant in excess then the receptor sites shut down almost entirely; this means you need more of the stimulant to get the same buzz as the original high. In practical terms, if one coffee lifts you up and you drink many cups a day, after a while you need a double espresso to achieve the same effect as the original regular coffee. It's like having to shout louder as you are speaking to ears that have become hard of hearing.

Gut Health

A human body is actually composed of more bacteria than cells. These trillions of bacteria are collectively called the microbiome, There is a large cluster of bacteria in our gut. They play a huge role not just in gut health, but overall health. In recent years research has shown that imbalance of gut bacteria (called dysbiosis) may contribute to neurological conditions including anxiety, Parkinson's disease and Alzheimer's disease. Jane Foster, an associate professor of neuroscience and behavioral science at McMaster University, Ontario, says gut bacteria 'talk to the brain in multiple ways through either the immune system or the enteric nervous system'.

Increasingly scientists are referring to the gut as a second brain, which has its own nervous system – the enteric nervous system. Traditional thinking is that the brain is 'in charge' of your body, however your gut sends far more information to your brain, via the vagus nerve, than your brain sends to your gut. Neurotransmitters are also made in the gut, so gut health directly influences how we feel.

A healthy diet, including natural probiotics and a good intake of digestive enzymes (found in uncooked plants and vegetables), helps to maintain and calm the gut. Healthy gut bacteria activate neurons in the brain that produce serotonin.

> *Antibiotics can delete the healthy bacteria. Taking*
> *a 28-day supplementation of probiotics after a*
> *course of antibiotics is highly recommended.*

Prebiotics are less well known and are specialized plant fibres that nourish the existing gut bacteria. While probiotics populate the gut with new bacteria, prebiotics feed them and sustain them. In this way they are equally as important for gut and brain health.

When I was a student of nutrition, we were taught to imagine our body as a Polo mint with a hole in the centre. Our body is the mint and our digestive system the hose that goes through the middle, running from our mouth to our anus. Quite a picture isn't it! But it's a useful analogy. However, our digestive system *does* interact with our body as, unlike a hose, it's totally permeable in places, so that nutrients and waste products can be picked up and transported. Digestion is such a complicated process so it makes sense that it has its own dedicated network of neurons to oversee it all.

As we have learnt much earlier, NT's carry messages across the synapse, but these messages have to be received in special receptor sites. These are made from essential fatty acids (EFAs), in particular phospholipids. Your body has the capacity to produce some phospholipids naturally, but you can also get phospholipids, including the lecithin vital for health (especially liver health and function), from dietary sources such as:

- Egg yolks
- Liver
- Wheat germ
- Peanuts.

You can also find phospholipids in:

- Soy
- Milk
- Lightly cooked meats
- Most fats, oils.

The best sources of EFAs are often referred to as 'The Magic Four':

1. Fish (oily, not farmed)
2. Nuts (fresh, uncooked)
3. Seeds (fresh, uncooked)
4. Eggs (Organic)

These four essential foods are vital for both a healthy brain and a healthy body.

They sharpen our memories, improve our moods and help keep us motivated. A good balance of EFAs is also essential to prevent cravings.

• •

Chapter 12

Fat Cells or Flat Cells?

Your fat cells — those things that store your fat and make you look flabby — are actually tiny, minute in fact. The size of a typical fat cell in an adult of a 'healthy weight' is about 0.6 micrograms (a microgram is one millionth of a gram, so fats cells are pretty small). However, they can expand. To what size depends on the individual, but it's estimated the maximum expansion is 0.9 micrograms. When they are full, fat cells have the ability to replicate, as happens in obese individuals.

The good news is that when they are empty, the minute size of fat cells means we don't look fat and flabby anymore! Some scientists now view fat cells as part of the endocrine system, because they aren't as dormant as was once thought — they produce oestrogen and other chemical messages. If protein is the building block of muscles, fat is the building blob of fat!

How to Shrink Your Fat Cells

I am going to keep this part quite brief. You are smart and you already know most of the key points I'm going to teach you now. But the foremost among them is this: *get moving*! If you want to burn fat, you *must* move your body. I told you earlier that the only place your body burns fat is in your muscles, so you *must* move and strengthen your muscles. Otherwise it would be like having a car in the garage that burns fat instead of petrol. If you never take it out of the garage, or only do short journeys, it burns very little fat, despite its potential!

Essentially, there are two types of exercise – aerobic and anaerobic. Aerobic simply means 'with oxygen'. Aerobic is the only system that burns fat. Three things need to combine to produce energy 'aerobically' – fat, oxygen and glucose. Fat cannot be burned on its own, which is a shame because otherwise you could just get up in the morning, go for a 10-hour walk and come home at the end of the day a stone lighter! Sadly, our bodies don't work like that. They just can't burn fat without oxygen and glucose. It's a simple law of physics. In the same way you can't light a fire without the presence of oxygen, within your cells you can't burn fat without oxygen and glucose. All three must be present for the combustion of the fat to take place.

Your aerobic capacity is entirely dependent on the ability of your cardiovascular system to pump oxygen (which is carried in red blood cells) around the body. If you have a weak heart and circulation system, your ability to exercise is restricted because you can't get the oxygen you need delivered to your muscles to move them. As you know from the previous chapter, glucose (from carbohydrate) is used *by every cell, all the time*. It is the primary source of energy for everyday functions. Your brain, in particular, has a dominant need for glucose, and as we have already seen, if levels within your body drop too low, you have a special in-built survival mechanism that literally breaks down your muscle tissue and converts it into glucose (producing ketones) to meet the brain's need for fuel. Critically, you do *not* need oxygen or anything else to burn glucose for energy.

Many diets (high-protein, low-carb based diets in particular) use this theory to achieve weight loss, i.e. restricting glucose supply so that, instead, you use fat to meet your energy needs, when in fact you cannot burn fat without glucose. As another function of glucose is to enable us to store water within our cells, the combined fluid and muscle loss can be quite drastic on the scales, but in reality you end up with a higher percentage of body fat even though you weigh less. You are lighter, but flabbier. As I explained in the last chapter, when glucose levels drop too low you compensate by metabolizing your own muscle, or lean body mass (LBM), which is the key factor in determining how many calories you are able to burn every day.

When you go back to 'normal' eating, you cannot physically burn as many calories as you did before because your LBM determines your metabolic rate – less LBM means a lower metabolic rate, so you not only regain any weight lost (usually as more fat), but gain extra fat as well. In this way it's very easy to use what is essentially a survival mechanism to diet yourself fat. Does this sound familiar? The answer is not to have so much glucose that you don't need to burn fat, but not too little that you need to cannibalize your muscle tissue to make up the deficit. It's all about balance.

A diet too high in protein and too low in carbs can also disrupt the body's natural balance, including its pH levels, which can lead to osteoporosis, kidney damage, heart disease and many other serious health consequences. Protein is important, essential in fact, but in the right quantities.

Getting the balance of nutrients right is what forms the basis of the colour-code system and you can be confident that all the calculations have been done for you. If you choose the right number of foods from the right colour groups, you will be nourishing your body, helping to balance your hormones, and enhancing your fat-burning capabilities.

Burning Fat

So, you now know that the key to effective fat burning is to ensure you have the right amount of glucose in your bloodstream to meet your body's needs, so that when challenged with activity or movement, it has to dip into your fat stores, which it then blends with the glucose and burns using oxygen. Every time you move your muscles, you are burning some fat; you are also burning some fat at rest, and even at night. When you sleep restfully, the hormones that promote fat burning are stimulated – the amount you burn is dependent on what you have eaten, how active you've been, your hormone levels and the amount of LBM you have.

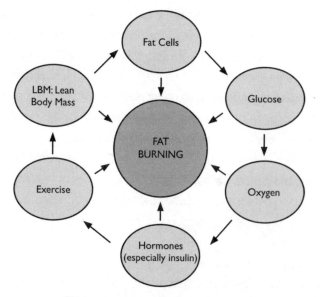

The key components of efficient fat burning

Every time you exercise, the hormones and enzymes that release and burn fat become more efficient. The growth and repair of your muscle tissue — which occurs overnight during restful sleep — builds healthier, stronger muscles — increasing your lean body mass (LBM). This enables you to burn more fat every day, even when you are not exercising.

Anaerobic means 'without oxygen'. Remember, you can burn glucose on its own without fat or oxygen (but not the other way around), and you do this in all cells except muscle cells, which use fat and oxygen as well as glucose. When you are weight training you are working anaerobically: you are loading one specific muscle group for a very short period of time. Let's say you are doing a leg press exercise in the gym. The exercise set may be over in less than a minute, so your body doesn't have time to send a message out to your fat cells, asking them to release the fat into your bloodstream and then direct it through the circulation system to your thigh muscles to mix with glucose and oxygen.

However, if you were to use your thigh muscles for power walking or cycling, then the workload would be much lower. After all, you can walk for a lot longer than you can do a heavy leg press, so you are much more likely to keep the activity going for longer. Now your body does have time to liberate fat from the cells, circulate it and get it to the working muscles on a constant basis.

Which Exercise Is Best?

In reality, we are always using a combination of both aerobic and anaerobic 'systems'. Humans are aerobic creatures — we cannot survive without oxygen — but as you learnt in the section on insulin, we also have the ability to switch energy systems according to the demands on our body and which fuel supplies we have available.

The difference is not dissimilar to that of comparing electricity with gas: if you walk into a cold room and you want instant energy, you put on an electric fan heater; if you want longer-term heat then you put on the central heating, which, although takes longer to work, is very efficient and can last for hours. Electricity is like using glucose alone — it's immediately available, whereas central heating is like mixing glucose with oxygen and fat — it takes longer to get going because it relies on a circulation system to be delivered, just like your radiators need hot water to be pumped from the boiler.

An aerobic activity such as power walking, jogging or cycling will become anaerobic as you get more tired and your heart has to work harder to supply the oxygen. At the beginning of a 30-minute workout, assuming you have warmed up correctly and raised your heart rate gradually, you will be working mainly aerobically. After about 15 minutes, if you are beginning to feel a little more challenged, the ratio will change slightly — you will be using less fat and oxygen as your circulation is struggling to keep up delivery, and relying more on glucose. If by the end of 30 minutes you are wiped out, you will be in your anaerobic zone (relying almost totally on glucose), which you can't sustain for more than a few minutes. This is when athletes 'hit the wall'. In a fit individual this takes a marathon to reach, but in a very unfit individual it can be reached after as little as a few minutes of activity.

In terms of burning fat, we have established that you burn fat when you work aerobically, *but* there is also an energy cost *after* you've finished exercising that also burns fat, and this is determined by the intensity of the workout. In simple terms, the harder you work out during your exercise session, the more fat you burn afterwards. So, comparing activities and how much fat they burn when you do them can be very misleading.

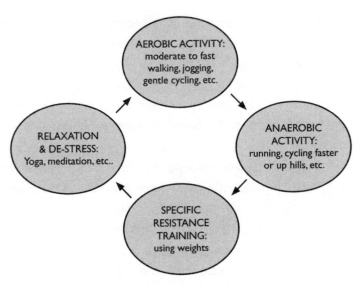

The key components of an effective exercise regime

Anaerobic exercise in particular has been shown to be beneficial for boosting thyroid function – specifically when working at 70 per cent or above of your maximum heart rate. So short bursts of intense activity, such as running and cycling (assuming you are fit enough) are beneficial as part of your overall exercise regime. This is something you can work up to gradually if your fitness levels are currently low. A mixture of high and low intensity exercise on different days will yield the best results.

Resistance training, i.e. with weights, will increase your metabolic rate so you burn more calories, even when you are not exercising. Resistance training increases your lean body mass (LBM), which is made up primarily of muscle. Always remember this: the *only* cells in your body that can burn fat are your muscle cells, so if you increase the strength and efficiency of your muscles (your LBM), your ability to burn fat increases, even when you are not exercising. This is so important it is worth repeating: *only muscles burn fat!*

Any exercise regime designed to promote fat loss *must* include some form of resistance exercise that will replace some of the natural muscle wastage that comes with age and inactivity. Every pound of muscle burns 40 calories per day at rest, so if you can increase your muscle density, your everyday fat-burning potential is drastically increased. This is why on some programmes there is a visible change in body composition – your clothes become looser and you look and feel better, but there is negligible weight loss on the scales because you are losing fat mass and building muscle (LBM). This does level out after a while, but as long as you are losing inches, and starting to look and feel better, don't worry if you are not losing as much weight as you think you should be. You are changing your body composition and that will lead to a long-term loss of fat.

Taking It Slowly

One client once told me she had been exercising regularly, had been 'really good' with her food, felt her clothes were getting looser, but when she went for her weekly weigh-in at her slimming club she was 'told off' for only losing half a pound. Totally demotivated, she immediately went home, ate six slices of toast and gave up.

Three years later, and now two stone heavier, she came to see me. This happens all the time and it's purely down to not understanding how the body works and responds to change. Always remember the story of the Three Little Pigs: the quickest way is not the best way and what looks good from the outside often doesn't last. If you are losing inches, then you are losing fat weight.

The primary goal is to get fit and healthy, so your hormones can function properly to allow you to burn fat. Depending on your start point – how out-of-balance your system is – it may take a few weeks for this to correct before you start to see significant weight loss. Be patient though, and focus on balancing your system first – when you do this, the weight will come off naturally.

Exercise

Write down three things in your journal you can do regularly that will increase your body's ability to burn fat:

1. ....

....

2. ....

....

3. ....

....

Then say each one out loud and with emotion.

One final point about exercise – for as many years as I can remember, the question I'm asked most about exercise is: 'Which is the best exercise for weight loss?' technically the answer is cross country skiing, but in reality the correct answer is: 'The exercise you most enjoy doing', because that's the only one you are likely to stick to.

When I'm asked, 'How hard should I work?' my answer is, 'As hard as you can for as long as you can, and as often as you can – depending on your fitness level'. That way you maximize the calories you burn when you work out, but also increase your metabolic rate on the days you are not working out. Keep in mind that relaxation and de-stressing should also make up part of your regime. Ideally, you will combine a mixture of different activities so you can work aerobically and also build LBM. Bear in mind when designing your activity or exercise regime that it has to be something you *enjoy*. Even a game of badminton twice a week or a Zumba class will burn calories and get you moving. So the bottom line is this: just do something!

....

Chapter 13

Food Matters

Earlier in the book I told you how, when I was researching my Master's degree dissertation, I wanted to show that if people record what they eat, they automatically choose healthier foods, and as a result, lose more weight. My results did show that, but I also found an unexpected benefit of teaching people about how to eat well – during the six weeks of the nutrition course that I ran prior to the actual study, the average weight loss was greater than in the 10 weeks that followed. Despite the fact that I'd asked my volunteers not to change what they ate until the study began, almost all of them made small changes that had a significant impact on their weight. Many of them lost a dress size without even consciously trying! It didn't help my study at the time, but it did teach me a valuable lesson that I have used to help many people since: Knowledge Is Power or, put another way, Awareness Is Curative.

Having proven that food recording is a helpful tool for achieving weight loss, I also realized that for most people, writing down everything you eat is a real pain. I wanted to create a system that made food recording simple, so I separated the main food groups into different colours, and simply asked people to make a note of how many portions of each colour they ate. Of course, I had to give them guidelines to follow about how many portions of each colour would be best. After two years of trialling different combinations and colours, and analyzing numerous diets, I created the colour-code system that you see in the next chapter. Since then I've continued to refine and improve it, and the system I'm bringing you now is, I believe, the very best way to follow a well-balanced 'diet', without actually dieting. You will get all the proven benefits of food recording, without the hassle. The Food Record cards take just a few seconds to complete – you simply tick the box of the colour of the food you are eating.

What Makes a Good 'Diet'?

Before we get into the colour-code system itself, let me give you an overview of it, and teach you a few key facts about nutrients – how they are digested and what your body needs nutritionally to be healthy *and* to burn fat.

The word 'diet' simply means what you eat – or scientifically speaking, 'your energy intake' (or EI). So in truth, we are *all* on a diet. It's the slimming diet mentality that's the problem, though, because it involves deprivation or avoidance – often of valuable nutrients – for the sole purpose of losing weight and with little or no regard for the long-term impact on our health. All that stops now!

It's currently very fashionable to base 'diets' on what our ancestors ate – specifically cavemen, who were hunter-gatherers. I find the fixation with eating the same as cavemen somewhat bemusing, because cavemen had a significantly shorter lifespan than we do. They were also probably extremely hungry a lot of the time, and had to eat what was available rather than choose their foods based on what tasted, smelt or looked good. There are, of course, elements of this 'diet' that are good, but not the complete concept. The reason cavemen were slim was due as much to the fact that they were highly active physically, and that their diets contained no high-fat, high-sugar foods, or indeed any excess of food. I really enjoy my food, so this sort of restrictive regime doesn't appeal to me one bit!

However, it is clear that when high-sugar, high-fat foods are unavailable, our diets are automatically much healthier. One example of this was seen in the period during and immediately after World War II, when rationing was in force. Meat was in short supply and people had to rely a lot more on homegrown vegetables. There are elements of this postwar 'deprivation' that would benefit us today. Engine fuel was also rationed, so although people didn't have to chase their dinners, they did have to walk everywhere instead of taking the car. It is no coincidence that the population at this time was slimmer and the incidence of heart disease was much lower.

The reality is that there are some good elements to most diets – it's just that they are so often taken to extremes. The high-protein diet, for example, was initially based on some sound concepts, but these were made so extreme that they became potentially very harmful to health, if sustained. Refined foods such as bread, rice or pasta are not allowed on the high-protein diet and it's recommended that lots of lean meat and fish be consumed. These elements of the diet are sound up to a point, but others – such as consuming little or no fruit – should be ignored. Doing that would be to deny your body the valuable antioxidant (cancer-preventive) nutrients that it simply must have, as well as the many phytochemicals and fibre these foods contain (more about this in the section on carbohydrates).

There seems to be a fixation with coming up with faddy, fashionable diets in which some obvious concepts are ignored for fear of being boring, or not 'sexy' enough to market. I will not bow to that pressure! Instead, I will give you the information you need, and then show you how to adapt the colour-code system to make it work for you. One thing's for sure, no more faddy dieting (and I'll leave the 'sexy' bit to you!!)

You *can* calculate approximately how many calories you need to consume on a daily basis, but unless you are going to count *every* calorie you eat, there's little point. In the colour-code system, if you stick to the guidelines and the portion sizes, you will probably be eating around 1,800 calories per day. If you are active, this is enough to lose weight and satisfy you at the same time. You may not even be able to eat this amount! However, you should *never* go below 1,500 calories per day, as this can result in a drop in your metabolic rate and reduce your capacity to burn fat.

Here in the Western world, our lifestyles have become increasingly sedentary, and this has impacted greatly on how much we need to eat. Our parents and grandparents were by necessity much more active than we are today. We need 30–50 per cent less energy than they did. This means that if we eat like they did, we'll get fat, and surprise surprise, we eat *even more* than they did, so we've got *really* fat!

Fats, Protein and Carbohydrates

Fats, protein and carbohydrates are the three main nutrients (excluding water) that your body needs to function. They work together to provide energy and on-going growth and repair. When eaten in the right amounts, and from the right sources, they provide us with protection from disease, slow down the ageing process, and give us vitality and longevity.

The amount of each nutrient that you need as an individual varies and is determined largely by your activity levels and your age. For example, athletes and more active people need more carbohydrates than sedentary people because they have a higher energy requirement – also weight loss is not an issue for them as most of the glucose they ingest is used up quickly and they don't have to worry about the fat-storing effects of high blood sugar.

There is no set figure for the exact amount or percentage of each nutrient you should have in your diet, and two individuals may function better on slightly different amounts, depending on various factors, but the graphic below gives you a general guideline:

**50%
CARBOHYDRATES**
Including vegetables,
crunchy fruit,
unrefined cereals
and grains

**50% FATS &
PROTEIN**
Including fish, lean
meat, eggs, beans
and pulses

Key nutrients and their optimum percentages within your diet

Fats

There are two types of fat:

1. **Saturated Fatty Acids (SFAs)** – solid at body temperature (37°C/98°F).

2. **Unsaturated Fatty Acids (UFAs)** – essential fatty acids or EFAs – liquid at body temperature.

Both contain nine calories per gram.

Fats should make up approximately 30 per cent of your diet. That does not mean that this percentage of your diet should be fish and chips, Chinese takeaways and ice cream, though! Getting the balance right between SFAs and UFAs is key.

Saturated Fatty Acids

SFAs are found in meat and animal products, including dairy. Chocolate is also a major source, and despite claims for its antioxidant properties, should be eaten in extreme moderation. An average bar of milk chocolate has approximately 9.1 grams of saturated fatty acids, which is 46 per cent of the RDA (Recommended Daily Allowance). Pure cocoa powder, on the other hand, has hardly any at all – less than one per cent. It's a good substitute for chocolate in baking, if you want to get the chocolate taste without the fat.

Other animal products that are high in saturated fatty acids include processed meats such as pâté, which is also combined with butter and in most cases cream, making it a very high-calorie food. Hard cheese and butter are also full of SFAs. The only two saturated fatty acids that do not come from animal sources are coconut oil and palm oil (more about the health benefits of coconut oil later on).

Put simply, saturated fats make you heavy and fat. If you want to consume the maximum amount of SFAs in one meal, then a lamb korma or passanda would be about as high as you can get – especially if you have it with a naan bread, because that is also very high on the glycaemic index or GI (*see page 229*). A naan bread alone contains more than 500 calories and would almost certainly be converted to fat; throw in a pint of beer or some wine and it would be difficult to find a heavier more fat-storing meal! A much healthier Indian meal would be chicken tikka or tandoori, with a vegetable curry side dish and a small portion of basmati rice or a chapati (not both!). With Chinese food, so much of it is fried that it's easy to consume lots of fatty and high GI foods. A good option there would be to have steamed fish with vegetables, and a small amount of boiled or steamed rice. If you stop yourself going to these kinds of restaurants you may feel like a bit of a pariah, socially. I love going for an Indian meal or getting a takeaway sometimes, but those are the type of dishes I choose. Remember the friend I told you about earlier who lost weight by 'Becoming a boring bas****'? This is exactly why you must still go out and do the things that you did before, just with a few modifications. When I go out, I don't have any less fun than my friends who eat lamb passanda, I just don't go home fatter!

In the first section of the book, you learnt about how your brain works and how important positive associations and emotions are, so it's *vital* that you learn to adapt the things you enjoy so you don't feel like you are on a diet. If you stop everything you like overnight, you are less likely to stick to the programme. In fact, I can almost guarantee you won't. Most meals, including trips to restaurants, can be managed with some careful choices and you won't have to drastically change your lifestyle.

SFAs – Friend or Foe?

Having some saturated fatty acids in the diet is acceptable; in fact if you are a meat eater, or enjoy hard cheese, then it's impossible not to get some. However, in the Western world most people consume far too many SFAs and not enough unsaturated fatty acids (UFAs), which has a huge and negative impact on our health. UFAs, and in particular the essential fatty acids omega-3 and omega-6, provide the structure for all cell membranes and are vital for good health. An excess of SFAs however, gets deposited in our fat stores and increases our risk of a whole range of diseases including heart disease, diabetes, stroke and cancer. Too much saturated fat is a killer. It looks bad from the outside and its effects are even worse on the inside.

Remember this: if a fat solidifies at room temperature (i.e. once it's out of the oven and cooled), it will solidify *inside* your body once digested. That's what makes it a saturated fatty acid. Think what your roasting tray looks like after you've cooked a joint of beef or lamb – there will be a sticky, white layer of fat in the bottom when it cools and that's exactly what will be happening inside your body when you've eaten it. The saturated fatty acids in meat have been stored there by the animal for the same reasons you store SFAs – for energy. So when you eat a lot of meat, it's not even *your* fat that's making you fat, you are getting 'ready-made' fat from the animal, who has done all the conversion for you!

Coconut Oil deserves special mention in this section as, in the past, it has been demonized as one of the only two saturated fats (the other is palm oil) that doesn't come from animals. However, research has shown that the fatty acids in coconut oil differ from animal fats and can be beneficial to health, especially brain function.

Some populations who live in remote areas are among the highest consumers of saturated fats in the world, and over 60 per cent of their calories come from coconuts, yet they enjoy good health, with little or no evidence of heart disease, as normally associated with SFAs. Coconut is the best oil for cooking as it is stable at high temperatures. If you buy a jar of organic coconut oil, you can also add a large handful to your moisturizer, or put it directly onto any areas of dry skin. Within a few weeks or less you will notice a real difference.

When it comes to the most easily recognizable sources of SFAs, I'm sure I don't need to tell you which foods not to eat – you are too smart for that. If I have to cover the next few pages with a list of crisps, chips, chocolates, cakes, fatty meats, pastries, cheesy pizzas and pies etc., then you are in serious denial. What I may need to tell you about is the fats that you *do* need to eat: the fats that improve your health by helping to balance your hormones and also aid your metabolism, therefore helping you to lose weight.

Unsaturated Fatty Acids

The key difference between the two types of fat is that unsaturated fatty acids (UFAs) are liquid at room temperature, and therefore within the body. This liquidity means they can be used for things like cell membranes – in fact every cell in your body has a membrane made of UFAs. However, the fact they are so delicate that they can be used in this way also makes them fragile, and exposure to heat, light or even oxygen reduces or eliminates their nutritional qualities. This is why you pay so much more for extra virgin cold-pressed olive oil – it has been extracted from the olive in a cold, darkened room to preserve its quality. Good quality oils like this always come in darker bottles to protect them further from the light and should be stored in a cool, dark place. When it comes to cooking, use them for dressings but never for cooking because heat not only destroys any nutritional benefit, it actually makes them toxic and harmful. Do add a few drops of extra-virgin oil to your roast potatoes or stir-fry *after* you've cooked them in vegetable or coconut oil though, as this gives them extra flavour.

While we need some SFAs for insulation and for energy, we don't need much. It's an area of controversy among nutritionists but a guideline would be to eat a ratio of two or three UFAs to one SFA. Unsaturated fatty acids can be broken down further into monounsaturated fatty acids (MUFAs) and polyunsaturated fatty acids (PUFAs); these are also called essential fatty acids (EFAs). We don't need to go into great detail here, but the difference between these is in the length of the carbon chain and how valuable and usable each is within the body. For our purposes we just need to know that you need *both*. You can see the foods that contain these different types of fat in the table opposite:

The unsaturated fatty acids in food (including the phospholipids mentioned earlier) are more easily absorbed than those found in supplements, so although supplements can be useful, they are not intended to be replacements for UFAs in the diet. If you want to be healthy and slim, you must look at your diet and make sure you are taking in the right materials to carry out the job of making you slim! One of the easiest ways to get a good balance of omega-6 and omega-3 is to crush some fresh seeds every morning and sprinkle them on cereal just before eating; or at some other time in the day, toss them in a salad. An ideal blend would be flax and pumpkin (omega-3), with sesame and sunflower (omega-6). Because it's easier to consume omega-6 in the diet, use twice as much flax and pumpkin. Alternatively, you can grind some hemp seeds – these already contain a good balance of both essential fatty acids. Hemp seeds are from the marijuana plant, but the seeds do not make you high and can be sold legally in a health food shop!

MONOUNSATURATED FATTY ACIDS	POLYUNSATURATED FATTY ACIDS (ESSENTIAL FATTY ACIDS, OR EFAS)	
	OMEGA-3	OMEGA-6
Olive oil (cold-pressed)	Oily fish	Evening primrose oil
Avocado	Flax seeds	Wholegrain, unrefined cereals
Peanut oil/butter	Pumpkin seeds	Eggs (fresh, organic)
Almond oil	Walnuts	Sunflower seeds
Canola oil	Soy beans	Poultry
	Green leafy vegetables	Most vegetable oils
		Hemp seeds (also good for Omega-3)
		Wholegrain bread
		Sesame seeds
		Soy beans
		Corn

Are You Getting Enough EFAs?

The benefits of unsaturated fats (including phospholipids), and in particular omega-3 and omega-6 are infinite in terms of your health. Rather than explain in detail what these essential fatty acids do, here's a list of some of the many symptoms of a deficiency of EFAs:

- Skin problems – especially dry skin conditions such as eczema
- Hair loss
- Liver degeneration

- Kidney degeneration
- Gland malfunction
- Susceptibility to infection
- Failure to heal
- Arthritis and other inflammatory conditions
- Heart and circulation problems
- Behavioural disturbances
- Growth retardation
- Impaired vision
- Tingling sensations in arms and legs
- Loss of coordination
- General inflammation
- High blood pressure
- High triglyceride levels (fats in the blood)
- Sticky platelets (causes clotting)
- Increased risk of cancer.

Some years ago I went to a seminar by Udo Erasmus, who is arguably the world's leading expert on fats. I was more than impressed by his delivery, and the way he explained the nature and importance of essential fatty acids in the diet was truly inspirational. If you think you may have an EFA deficiency, or would like more information on the scientific nature of EFAs and other nutrients then I would recommend his book, *Fats That Heal, Fats That Kill*. If I could only ever own one nutrition book, this would be it. It is the absolute 'fat bible'!

If you suffer from any of the more serious conditions listed above, or in particular, if you have ever suffered from cancer, then the information you need to regain health is beyond the scope of this book, but Udo's book, and his range of oils, are absolutely essential for you. Visit www.udoschoice.co.uk for more information, and to see a range of his outstanding products.

By using the colour-code system in Chapter 12, you will learn how to choose the right foods to ensure that you get a good intake of EFAs, and enjoy all the health benefits that entails. If you have been deficient for some time, it can take several weeks, or in extreme cases even months, to see visible changes on the exterior (skin), because the cells inside will always heal first. Once again, I remind you of the man who chose the penny and sat back and enjoyed his compound interest!

Protein

Contains four calories per gram.
Protein is the element of food that gives it – and us when we eat it – structure. It is contained in meat and animal products, but also in non-animal foods such as seeds, nuts and all pulses. Protein should make up approximately 20–25 per cent of your total dietary/ daily intake. It is a vital component of all living cells. After water, protein is the most abundant nutrient in our bodies, but despite its importance, the reason you need less protein than carbohydrate or fat is because, unlike the other fats and carbs, protein is not used for energy production. Therefore it doesn't need to be replaced as often because it stays in the body for much longer.

Protein is made up of amino acids, which are like building blocks. If we put them together in the right way, we can make whatever we need for our bodies out of these blocks. Think of it this way: we have 26 letters in our alphabet, which we use in different combinations to make up all the words we need, but to make a word, we need to include a vowel to give it structure. In the same way, we use a variety of amino acids to build healthy cells and structures, but we must include one of the eight *essential amino acids* in order to make a complete structure.

There are a few fundamental differences in the way the body handles protein compared to fat or carbohydrates. Protein takes a long time to digest and therefore keeps us satisfied for a long time, whereas carbohydrate digestion begins in the mouth. Protein can only be digested in the stomach because it's much harder to break down. The stomach is a sealed sac that contains a special acid called hydrochloric acid that is required to break down protein. The stomach lining is covered in a coating of thick, phlegm-like fluid that protects it against the harmful effects of the acid. If the acid does escape to other areas outside the stomach, it causes burns and ulcers, so there are valves at the entrance and exit of the stomach to prevent this from happening. Both fat and carbohydrates need to pass through the stomach to be digested in the intestines, as they need different alkaline enzymes to break them down.

How Much Protein Is Enough?

There has been a lot of controversy in recent years about the benefits, or otherwise, of the 'high-protein, low-carb' diet – and the many other diets that are variations on the same theme. As you know, certain aspects of this regime are helpful, but if taken to extremes, they can be terribly harmful. Protein contains nitrogen, which the body converts into ammonia and then urea; this is excreted by the kidneys. This highly acidic process can be undertaken safely while the correct amount of protein is being eaten, but if the diet is consistently high in protein the kidneys can begin to suffer from the effects of the extra work they need to do. This can be felt as anything from a slight backache to – at worse – full kidney failure.

A long-term, high-protein diet has other potentially serious negative effects. For example, the body becomes too acidic and, to combat this, it extracts calcium (which is very alkaline) from the bones and dumps it into the bloodstream to compensate. Over time, this can lead to osteoporosis, as well as an increased risk of heart disease, because circulating calcium makes the blood very viscous (scratchy) and can damage artery walls. High-protein diets also prohibit the intake of fruits and vegetables (which is *not* a good thing); although they do also limit high-GI refined carbs (which *is* a good thing).

In the previous chapter, we looked at why you need to increase the amount of muscle tissue (LBM) in your body in order to maximize the amount of fat you can burn. However, eating vast amounts of protein does *not* do this. Your body decides how much protein to use for muscle growth (as opposed to many other things) based purely on how often and how much you use your muscles. If you sat on your bed and consumed vast numbers of protein shakes, you would still get fat.

Your body is smart – it has an intelligence beyond comprehension. It operates solely on feedback, so if your muscles are not sending messages to your brain saying, 'I need to be stronger', then no extra protein will be delivered for muscle growth. If, however, you are exercising and challenging your muscles *and* eating good quality protein, then your muscles, and therefore your metabolic rate, will increase.

In terms of diet, the problem is that many foods that contain protein also contain fat. This is why, as you will see, they are grouped together on the colour-code system. In fact, there are very few foods that contain protein that don't also contain fat (specifically oils and butter). Relying solely on meat to get your protein is not a healthy way to eat a balanced diet. Whether you are a vegetarian or a meat eater, you must ensure that you consume vegetables and grains and non-meat sources of good quality protein such as the following:

- Beans
- Lentils
- Fresh, uncooked seeds
- Fresh, uncooked nuts
- Wholegrains
- Low-fat dairy products (preferably organic).
- Quinoa (a grain/fruit from South America)
- Soya (e.g. tofu)

Carbohydrates

Contain four calories per gram.

A carbohydrate is simply any food that contains glucose. This may mean it's almost entirely glucose, or that it contains glucose and other nutrients. The easiest way to define a carbohydrate is that 'it doesn't have a face'. In other words, it's grown in or on the soil and doesn't come from animals. Years ago, carbohydrates were defined as 'simple' or 'complex' – this simply referred to the size of the molecules. We have now developed a much better understanding of the molecular make-up of carbohydrates and how they behave in our bodies.

Carbohydrates as a food group contain many different substances, including:

- Glucose
- Fructose (fruit sugar)
- Vitamins

- Minerals
- Fibre
- Phytochemicals
- Enzymes
- Prebiotics.

When we talk about carbohydrates we usually think first of glucose and 'sugar'. We've already explored the importance of maintaining healthy blood sugar levels, and understanding how we use glucose for energy: in this section we are going to look specifically at the foods that enable you to achieve and maintain the right blood glucose levels.

Sugar

There are two main kinds of sugar, although technically anything that ends in 'ose' is a sugar, we will focus on glucose, which is an immediately usable form of energy – and fructose (fruit sugar) – which has to be taken to the liver and converted to glucose before it can be used for energy. This is a crucial difference, because glucose raises blood sugar instantly and fructose has a more moderate effect. When your blood sugar i.e. glucose levels are too high, the excess is converted into body fat. When your fructose levels are too high, because fructose in processed in the liver, it creates fatty deposits inside the liver.

Eating foods with added fructose can raise blood sugar levels above normal, but the fructose you eat direct from fruit will not cause this if it is consumed as part of a healthy diet. The problem arises when it's added to refined foods. We are perfectly capable of digesting fructose, especially as it is combined with other nutrients and fibre, meaning it takes longer to reach the liver than glucose, which can be absorbed instantly into the blood stream from the tongue.

All sugars have a calorific value of 4 calories per gram; the same as protein, and less than half the calories of fat, which has 9 calories per gram. Providing you eat low GI foods (see below), you can eat more food in terms of weight and yet eat fewer calories. However, because it's so easy to overeat refined, fat-free or fat-reduced foods, you can easily eat twice as much as you would do if the food contained fat. This is why so many people struggle to lose weight on the low-fat diet.

I can't tell you how many food diaries I have seen over the years that were virtually fat free, but where the individual was eating so much fat-free food that they overcompensated for the fat calories they had removed with starchy carbohydrates or sugars. They would have a huge plate of pasta with only a tiny amount of Bolognese sauce because they saw the pasta as fat-free, therefore not fattening. Some had been told by certain slimming clubs to eat meringues, which are almost 100% sugar, as they were 'low fat'. They ate so much fat-free pasta, rice, bread (without butter) and sugary foods that it caused a massive glucose spike and their bodies released extra insulin to convert the excess to fat. They got fat without even eating fat! Although ironically they thought they were 'being good'.

Fibre

This is worth a special mention as many of the best carbohydrates are high in fibre. This valuable nutrient aids transit time, i.e., the time it takes for a food to get from your mouth, have the nutrients extracted and pass out the other end. Slow transit time is a sign of a poor digestive system. I often ask clients how often they open their bowels and they say, 'Regular as clockwork – once or twice.' I say, 'That's great, twice per day?' and they say, 'No – once or twice per week.' They then proceed to tell me that their doctor tells them this is normal. It might be normal but it's certainly not desirable! You should open your bowels every day, more than once. If you are putting three meals in, you need to get three meals out, with the nutrients removed. If you are not then this must be addressed. I have covered this in the colour-code system. You will find that when you open your bowels more, you will be losing weight. Fibrous vegetables include prebiotics (important to help maintain healthy gut bacteria). A high protein diet excludes many foods high in fibre – yet another reason to avoid it.

The Glycaemic Index (GI)

GI is an invaluable tool. It's simply an index, or a list, that assigns to a food a numerical value that represents how quickly it is absorbed into the bloodstream. The key to understanding GI is to be aware that it determines the rate of digestion – it's that simple. Foods that speed quickly through your digestive system (such as refined foods) don't suppress appetite, whereas foods that reach the small intestine before they are fully digested (such as fibre-rich foods) stimulate the secretion of messenger signals to the brain saying, 'full up!' and you naturally stop eating because the hunger signal is switched off.

What you eat (not just how much) affects your appetite; if you stay fuller longer, then you are less susceptible to cravings and generally eat less. If you choose foods that are medium or low GI then you are assured of eating foods that take longer to digest and help suppress hunger. In addition, nature has given us another benefit associated with these foods: they are often rich in nutrients and contain many other vital components, including vitamins, minerals and fibre. When it comes to 'filling power', all foods are not equal, and that's what the GI helps us to understand.

Dr Jennie Brand-Miller is an Australian nutritionist known as 'The Queen of the Glycaemic Index', and the excellent book she co-authored, *The Low GI Diet*, led to a deluge of copycat diets and books. In a similar way to what happened with the high-protein diet, many of these took a sound concept to extremes. I have had clients come to me saying they are 'not allowed' to eat fruit. This is absolutely not true.

All About Antioxidants

The colour-code system in the next chapter takes full account of the principles of the GI. You will see that there are two classifications for carbohydrates: **PINK(P)** being the higher GI starchy foods that should be eaten in moderation (or some not at all!) and **GREEN(G)** which represents fruit and vegetables – these can be eaten freely.

Many people mistakenly stop eating fruit, thinking it causes a rush in blood sugar, but this is not the case as sugar in fruit – or, as we explained earlier, fructose – goes to the liver first before it can be used. There are very few exceptions to this rule – such as dates, some grapes, and melons – but if you eat these as part of a fruit salad with more fibrous fruit, they don't pose a problem. You would need to eat a very large portion of grapes to cause an insulin spike.

Fruits and vegetables are also an essential source of antioxidants; these are precious substances that protect against cancer and also slow down the ageing process. You don't have to be an expert to learn which foods contain antioxidants; there is a very simple guideline:

If it's fresh and colourful, it contains antioxidants.

The good news is that foods containing antioxidants are also typically low GI. For example, sweet potatoes are much lower on the GI than white potatoes, and are also rich in antioxidants.

Other foods high in antioxidants include the following:

- Carrots
- Broccoli
- Cabbage
- All berries: strawberries, cranberries, etc.
- Peppers (all colours)
- Watercress
- Cauliflower
- Melon
- Spinach
- Peas
- Tomatoes
- Lemons.

• •

Chapter 14

The Colour-code System

You are finally here! Now you know how your brain and body work, this section is the final piece of the puzzle. My goal is to give you enough nutritional information for you to be able to create a 'diet' that works for you and to make it as easy as possible to put into practice. The simple colour-code system that follows is designed to focus on getting you healthy and balancing your hormones so you become a natural fat burner. With this system *you* get to choose the foods you eat and you can create your own diet based on what you know will work. There are of course guidelines and suggestions but, unlike most diets, it is not a strict regime. As you know by now, no two people are exactly the same, so, based on how you feel, and how much weight you want to lose, you can adapt it slightly to find the right combination for you. Get this right and make the changes you are happy with and this *will* be the last 'diet' you will ever need.

You will find the guidelines for the Healthy Quick-Start Two-Week Plan in Chapter 15 (see *page 249*). This is a <u>*totally optional*</u> two-week programme that is simply a stricter version of the colour-code system. I have included this purely as an option as it has two benefits. Firstly, you give your liver and other systems a real boost, which will give you a head start in terms of making the physiological changes that are necessary to turn you from a fat storer to a fat burner; secondly, because it's always nice to see results quickly. We know that this activates our pleasure centres and as long as we enjoy what we are doing, we link pleasure to it longer term.

A WORD OF CAUTION

If, when you read about it, you feel like the Healthy Quick Start is too much like a diet, DON'T DO IT! You must only build positive associations with all the changes you are going to make now, so that you can change for good. After everything you have learnt, if you then go and follow a regime that you find hard and makes you feel deprived, you are in danger of undoing the good work you have already started.

I have three 'golden rules' when it comes to food:

1. **Never use any food as a reward or a treat.** Eat for one reason only: because your body needs fuel. And give it the best quality fuel possible. If you enjoy consuming the fuel, then so much the better! Eating is a great social activity and should be enjoyed, but eating out doesn't have to mean getting fat – you can apply my guidelines wherever you are.

2. **Never ban yourself from eating something.** This will only make you want it more. That doesn't mean I'm not going to say, 'don't have' certain foods – in a few cases I'm going to say just that! But I'm talking in general terms, and of course what I'm really saying is, 'If you have these foods other than once in a blue moon, you will get heavier or stay fat.' You make the final choice as to what you put in your mouth, not me.

3. **If you don't like it, don't eat it** – no matter how healthy or good for you it is! Make only positive food association.

The colour-code system is made up of four food groups. You will find a poster of each of the food groups in your journal. I encourage you to print these off and, for the first few weeks, stick them on your fridge or cupboard door to increase your awareness and remind you. Even better, you could make a collage or vision board of your own, using images of the foods that you love instead of my selection.

Green **G**

7–10 portions per day. Aim for minimum 2 per meal.

Vegetables and fruit and most foods (excluding starchy carbs) that grow in the soil. Range from medium–low GI, with a high nutritional content (including antioxidants); they also contain good levels of fibre.

Pink **P**

*1–3 portions per day. Aim for 1, maximum 3, per day and stick to recommended portion sizes. Always combine with a **B**.*

Starchy carbohydrates – i.e. all grains and related products (pasta, bread, rice, cereals, etc.) plus potatoes. Range from high–moderate GI foods with a moderate–good nutritional value, to high GI foods with a low nutritional value.

Blue **B**

Up to 5 portions per day (various sizes). Have 1–2 with each meal and use as snacks.

Fats and proteins, including fish, meat, dairy, nuts, seeds, oils. Range from high-nutritional-value foods containing good levels of EFAs to low-nutritional-value saturated fatty acids.

Red 🆁

Optional, irregular snacks.

Sweets, cream, ice cream, alcohol, sugar, refined honey, pastries (sweet or savoury), cakes, crisps, deep-fried chips, high-fat takeaway meals, etc. Food that has no nutritional benefit whatsoever – just empty calories.

In some of the groups, you will see a * beside a food. This indicates that it also contains strong elements of another group. For example, lentils are classified as 🅖 because they grow as beans in the soil and are a good source of fibre. When they are harvested and the lentils are separated from the plant, they are low on the glycaemic index. But they are also an excellent source of protein 🅑 so they cross two food groups. Another example is dried fruit, which is also 🅖, but has a higher GI than fresh fruit as much of the flesh and fluid has been removed, leaving mainly glucose; this has a *🅟 next to it.

You can use the arrows to gauge which foods are the best choice; wherever possible, reduce or avoid the choices at the bottom of the arrows and choose instead from the foods higher up the list.

How Much Should You Eat?

Each section/colour has an individual guideline for portion sizes. *How much* you eat is as important as *what* you eat. Remember I told you about all the low-fat dieters who got fat? Many of them ate more calories than they needed just because they weren't fat calories. You must become more aware of just how much you eat – even 'healthy' calories will make you fat if you eat too many of them.

You must use your own common sense and intelligence here. After all, you'll be kidding yourself if you think you can carry on eating as much as you are now and lose weight. It's also important to note that the speed at which you eat influences how *much* you eat.

Studies have shown that people who chew their food more, and who put their cutlery down in between each mouthful, eat less overall (estimates show this can be up to 200 calories less per meal!). Other studies have shown that if you eat in the dark (blindfold), then you have to pay more attention to the signals from your stomach to your brain and you stop eating much earlier. Using your eyes can literally by-pass this natural but subtle process.

Here is a great exercise to increase communication between your stomach and your brain and increase awareness of how full you are:

Exercise: The 10-Minute Rule

Before you start your meal, take a good look at the amount of food on your plate. Your stomach can comfortably distend to twice the size of your fist, so make a fist and put it next to your plate to give you a reference. Bear in mind, once inside your stomach it will have been chewed up. When over half way through a meal, close your eyes, draw your attention inwards and connect with your stomach. Visualize it and practise paying attention to how full it is. In between each mouthful put your mouth and fork down until you have chewed and swallowed. Every 10 mouthfuls close your eyes, go inwards and notice how your stomach feels. Stop eating as soon as you notice a sense of comfortable satisfaction. Wait 10 minutes, then go inside and notice if you feel even more satisfied (you almost certainly will as it can take several minutes to distend the stomach after each mouthful).

* *

Be aware that a portion size isn't designed to make you feel 'full up' – it's designed to satisfy and nourish you. There's a big difference between being satisfied, i.e. eating enough, and being full up. When you are full up, the uncomfortable sensation you get is your stomach telling you it is over-distended (stretched). Unfortunately, people get used to this sensation and programme themselves, or anchor it, to be the feeling they think they should get after every meal, and they don't stop eating until they get it. Next time you feel uncomfortable after eating, think about how much you've had and make a mental note to concentrate on how you feel internally, listen to your body and feel the signals. If you overeat for 10 minutes, you can consume an awful lot of calories you didn't need. The 10-minute rule can take inches off your waistline.

You can do this by understanding how the 'feedback' system between your stomach and your brain works. Your stomach has sensors all around it that send messages to the brain depending on how much it is distending. When you are tuned in to this sensation, your brain uses this signal to turn off hunger. Unfortunately, the sensation can be quite subtle and it's easy to ignore, especially if you eat quickly. By the time you process the signal you've already eaten overeaten and it's too late. Imagine your stomach as an empty balloon, but with a thick elastic band around it. As you blow the balloon up, the elastic band becomes tighter and you can see the amount of air that you can comfortably put into the balloon before the elastic band snaps. If your stomach snapped like the elastic band when you over-filled it, you'd be in trouble! Unlike the balloon though, your stomach can be severely overstretched before you physically have to stop eating.

TIP

Try this visual reminder to stop yourself from overeating. Wear a brightly coloured elastic band every time you eat to remind yourself that your stomach can carry on stretching long after you have had enough to eat. I've often given new clients a band and asked them not to take it off for two weeks (except to sleep). It's a simple technique but it has worked for many people – why not try it and see if it works for you.

Green Ⓖ

Cruciferous (leafy) green vegetables

All raw vegetables (including peppers)

Lightly cooked (or steamed) vegetables

Avocados *Ⓑ also a good source of EFAs

Lentils *Ⓑ also a good source of protein

Beans *Ⓑ also a good source of protein

Tofu *Ⓑ also a good source of protein

Frozen peas

Corn

All crunchy, not over-ripe fruit (e.g., apples and pears)

Soft fruits (including bananas) and berries

Fruit juice (unsweetened)

Dried fruit *Ⓟ high GI

Ⓖ *Portion Sizes*

All portion sizes given are guidelines, as individual body mass determines how many calories you need.

- Raw vegetables – unlimited
- Cooked vegetables – up to a large mug full
- Fruit: hand-held, e.g. bananas, apples, pears, oranges, etc. – one piece; except for avocado where half a fruit is one portion
- Berries – 2–3 heaped tablespoons
- Lentils/beans – I cup full (uncooked)
- Fruit juice – approximately 250ml (9fl oz): best diluted with water
- Dried fruit – small, level palm full (best eaten with something from Ⓑ group, such as nuts)

General Ⓖ *Guidelines*

- Eat I–2 portions of soft fruit per day.
- Eat as many different, brightly coloured vegetables and fruits as possible, e.g. green/orange/yellow/red – this will ensure a good balance of vitamins and minerals, as well as maximizing your intake of antioxidants.
- Dilute concentrated (unsweetened) fruit juice with water.
- Use raw spinach and watercress in salads rather than just lettuce leaves.
- Reduce the amount of meat you use in dishes such as curries and casseroles and replace with vegetables, beans or lentils. For example, make a chicken and vegetable curry in place of a chicken curry.

- Total portions from the **G** section per day: 7–10 (minimum 4 veg).

Pink

Quinoa

Barley

Oats

Brown rice/wild rice (al dente)

Basmati rice (al dente)

Sweet potato

Chickpeas

Muesli (no added sugar)

Couscous

Unrefined cereals (no added sugar)

Multigrain breads (with 'bits')

Rye bread

Fruit loaf

Wholemeal pasta (al dente)

White pasta (al dente)

Rye crispbreads

Chapatis

Gluten-free bread

Rice cakes

Wholemeal pitta bread

Corn wraps

Tortilla wraps

Brown bread

White pitta bread

Polenta

Bagels

Muffins

White bread

White potato

Unrefined honey

Waffles

Pizza

Sugar* (empty calories)

🅿 *Portion Sizes*

All portion sizes given are guidelines, as individual body mass determines how many calories you need.

- Quinoa, oats, rice, pasta, polenta, couscous, etc. – 1 cup full (uncooked)

- Sweet potato – 1 medium

- White potato – 1 medium or 4–5 small new potatoes

- Bread (including fruit loaf) – 2 medium-cut slices (multigrain) or 1 chapati

- Bagels/pitta breads/waffles/muffins/wraps, etc. – 1

- Unrefined honey and brown sugar – 1 teaspoon

- Cereals – 1 small bowl muesli (weight varies depending on ratio of ingredients: nuts are heavier than oat flakes), plus added fruit (any kind)

- Processed cereals – 250g (9oz)

- Crispbreads/rice cakes – 2

- Sugar/honey – 1 teaspoon

General 🅿 Guidelines

- 2–3 portions of 🅿 per day is fine as long as you choose from the top of the arrow, i.e. the lower GI options. If you are diagnosed, or suspect, you are insulin resistant or have problems balancing your blood sugar, halve the recommended portions sizes.

- Avoid or reduce the foods listed at the base of the arrow (i.e. from muffins and below).

- You must not exclude 🅿 altogether, as without them it's difficult to get the amount of glucose your cells need. The key is to choose the right ones (i.e. the ones at the top of the arrow).

- Total portions of 🅿 foods per day: 1–3.

Blue B

Fish (raw or lightly cooked and if possible, wild not farmed)

Udo's Oil (use in salad dressings or as a supplement)

Lean meat (preferably organic)

Fresh, uncooked nuts

Fresh, uncooked seeds

Extra-virgin olive oil

Eggs (organic if possible)

Cow's milk (organic if possible)

Rice milk

Almond milk

Soy milk

Yoghurt (low sugar)

Soft cheese

Hard cheese

Vegetable oils (for cooking)

Butter

Margarine

B Portion Sizes

Of all the food groups, the portion sizes vary more with B (fats and proteins) than any other colour. This makes sense when you look at the range of foods included, many of which contain fat and/or protein. The portion may be as small as some milk in your tea, or as big as a steak for your dinner! So you obviously need to exercise some common sense when choosing from this group. All sizes are guidelines, because individual body mass determines how many calories you need.

- Meat and fish – women 115–170g (4–6oz); men 170–225g (6–8oz)

- Fresh, uncooked nuts – a palm full

- Fresh, uncooked seeds (crack the husks before eating to release the oils) – 1 dessert spoonful

- Oils – 1–2 teaspoons per serving, e.g. in dressings mixed with vinegar

- Milk (all kinds) – approximately 250ml (9fl oz)

- Eggs – 1 large

- Yoghurt – 1 small pot

- Soft cheese 55–115g (2–4oz) as part of main meal or up to 55g (1–2oz) as a snack

- Hard cheese 55–115g (2–4oz) as part of main meal or up to 55 g (1–2oz) as a snack

- Butter – use sparingly

- Margarine – use sparingly

General **B** Guidelines

- Have a **B** food with every meal – it will keep you satisfied for longer.

- Do not eat only **B** foods – i.e. a high-protein diet. Always combine your overall intake of blues with **G** and/or **P** foods.

- Have meat no more than once per day (and have two meat-free days per week).

- Choose low-fat options wherever possible – including lean meat and skimmed or semi-skimmed milk and dairy produce.

- Hard cheese has much more saturated fatty acids than soft cheese, so moderate the amount of hard cheese you eat and mix with softer options.

- Use soft, lower-fat cheeses for making sauces, or choose a very strong hard cheese so you need only a little to get the cheesy taste you require.

- Watch out for low-fat options in the supermarket – they are often full of sugar to replace the taste of the fat.

- If you are vegetarian, you need to pay particular attention to the quality of the blues selected and not rely solely on cheese and other dairy products for your protein. Revisit the **G** section and look at beans, pulses and lentils, which also have a **B** star: you should have at least 1–2 portions of these per day.

- Use blues as part of your snacks, i.e. fresh uncooked nuts and seeds.

Red **R**

These are all the foods that have little or no nutritional value. It's not possible to list every single unhealthy food here, so once again use your common sense and don't deceive yourself!

All confectionery

Potato crisps

Chips

Pastries (sweet or savoury)

Alcohol

Canned, sugary drinks

High-fat takeaway meals

Cream/ice cream

Most cakes and biscuits

General Colour-Code System Guidelines

Let's make it really clear: *you are not on a diet!* So that means nothing is 'forbidden' and it's OK to have *anything* on the **R** list *sometimes*; that is occasionally, *not* every day. Now you have already learnt – and you can re-learn as you reread the chapters that have helped you the most – that with a combination of changing your mind, and what you eat, cravings can literally disappear. Your desire for unhealthy foods can and will diminish at your command!

The problem with these **R** foods is that you don't see the fat immediately after you eat them; so one takeaway doesn't mean you can't get into your jeans the next day. This is how we allow ourselves to overeat, because we cannot see the damage quickly enough to fully associate it with the foods we eat. However, you have now accepted that what you ate made you fat. I know you have, otherwise you wouldn't have got to this part of the book. So give yourself a huge pat on the back, and one from me!

If you find that you are having some **Ⓡ** foods every day, then go back and reread the chapters that you feel are the most relevant to you. As a very general guideline, aim to eat no more than 2–3 **Ⓡ** foods per week *maximum*. Please remember, though, that **Ⓡ** foods are not compulsory and this is the only colour group that it's OK not to have any of!

Use the information in both the psychological and nutrition parts of the book to achieve your goal. This really is a *mind and body approach*, and no other system has ever fully offered that, so make the most of all you have learnt and choose to make the changes that will give you the healthy body that is your birthright. Go and claim it now!

Chapter 15

Everyday Eating

In an ideal world, we would all have a wonderful and plentiful supply of organically farmed, fresh vegetables, and plenty of time off work to relax and de-stress, but for so many of us (I include myself!) that is not the case. So, we have to do the best we can with what we have. Nutritionally, you have a lot of great food available and by buying as much fresh produce as possible, limiting the amount of refined foods you eat, and using the colour-code system as your guide, you can look forward to a healthy, slim body and loads more energy.

Putting It All Together

Remember this key fact – you are not on a diet! But you do have to eat for the rest of your life, right? That means you need a system – a way of choosing the right foods that will last you a lifetime. This is that system; welcome to the colour-code system. I must emphasize again that *you* must take responsibility for what you eat: it's just not possible to design one 'diet' that works for absolutely everyone. But you can use the colour code template to create a lifetime eating plan that will bring you health and energy.

As a basic overview, if you aim for 2 **G**, 1–2 **B** and a maximum 1 **P** (or no pinks) in each meal, then you will be right on track. For snacks, stick to **G** and **B**.

There are moderate GI **P** options that should always be chosen in preference to the higher GI foods:

HIGH GI	MODERATE GI ALTERNATIVE
White potatoes	Sweet potatoes, yam, sweetcorn, beans, barley, lentils, chickpeas, soya beans (including tofu)
White rice	Quinoa, basmati rice, brown rice, vermicelli rice noodles, cellophane noodles (the clear ones)
Cereals (refined or processed)	Porridge oats, muesli (sugar-free)
White pasta	Wholewheat pasta (cooked al dente)
Canned spaghetti	Reduced-sugar tinned baked beans
White bread	Multigrain and seeded bread, fruit loaf, chapatis (made with chickpea flour, not wheat), wholemeal wraps

Fat and protein have no GI value and are therefore digested more slowly. This means if you combine something from these food groups (for example some brazil nuts – **B** on the colour-code system with a higher GI food such as a banana **G**, then the overall effect on your digestive system is influenced by the *combined* content of both foods.

Here are some other examples of how this works:

MODERATE GI	EAT WITH	PROTEIN/FAT
Jacket sweet potato	+	Tuna or soft cheese filling
Pasta (wholewheat)	+	Lean meat and/or vegetable sauce
Multigrain bread	+	Hummus or mashed avocado
Oats (cereal)	+	Yoghurt
Rice (basmati)	+	Mixed bean curry/casserole
Couscous	+	Meat or bean-based sauce

So it can be really simple. For a main meal, just choose a good quality protein such as lean meat, fish or beans **B**, eat with plenty of lightly cooked vegetables **G** and restrict the starchy GI foods to the lowest possible available – have no more than one **P** serving of starchy foods at any one time and if you have problems managing blood sugar, have half a serving. You don't need to eliminate pinks altogether. The moderate/low GI options are good brain fuel.

For snacks, do not have high GI or refined foods – stick to fruit and nuts, or raw vegetable nibbles (crudités) with some low-fat dips such as hummus.

The Daily Record Cards

I have mentioned several times how beneficial it can be to keep a record of what you eat. As you know, in my own studies I found this to be the case, but I also found that having to write everything down is a real nuisance and inconvenience. Everything I have taught you has been to avoid a regime that feels like a diet, so I created the Daily Record Cards to help you easily monitor what you are eating without having to weigh, measure and write it all down.

Below is an example of a Daily Record Card. You will also find a template in the back of your journal.

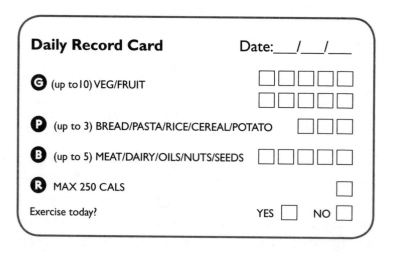

As you can see, each food group is followed by a series of boxes. Simply tick a box each time you have a food from that particular colour. By the end of the day you will be able to assess at a glance how many of each group you have eaten. It's up to you how long you use these cards for. In Chapter 3 you learnt about the process of change – starting with Conscious Competence, just like when you first learnt to drive and had to think about every manoeuvre, and after a while progressing to Unconscious Competence, i.e. driving along safely without even thinking about what you are doing.

If you are changing what you eat massively, you may need to use the Daily Record Cards for at least a month, or until your choices become second nature and you know you are on track without having to monitor it. If you have fewer changes to make, then you may only need to use them for a week or so. As with all of this programme, you must choose what works for you. Using these cards will accelerate your learning to the Unconscious Competence stage more quickly; you will be creating and saving brand new neurological maps. Even when you are on track, you can use them again, any time you feel you need a refresher. Even now, I still fill in a Daily Record Card to show at my seminars, and it never fails to get me focused.

Everyday Eating – Meal Suggestions

Breakfast

- Blend berries (fresh or frozen) **G** with yoghurt **B** and a spoonful of Udo's Oil **B**
- Muesli **P** with yoghurt or milk **B** and chopped fresh fruit **G**
- Porridge **P** with fruit **G** and a spoonful of seeds **B**
- SynerProTein drink (see *supplements section, page 268*) – in balance
- Fresh fruit salad **G** with yoghurt, nuts and seeds **B** and a spoonful of Udo's Oil **B**
- Baked beans **G** on multigrain toast **P** with a poached egg **B**
- Bacon **B**, poached eggs **B** and baked beans **G**

Lunch

- Sandwiches or wraps **P** filled with the following:
- Lean meat **B** with dark green salad leaves (i.e. spinach, rocket, watercress), tomatoes and cucumber **G**
- Brie **B** with beetroot **G**

- Tuna or salmon **B** with dark green salad leaves and tomatoes **G**
- Hummus **B**/**G** with dark green salad leaves and tomatoes **G**
- Vegetable soups (see *recipes, page 256*) **G**
- Baked beans **G** or poached eggs **B** on toast **P**
- Organic peanut butter **B** on toast **P** with sliced apple **G**
- Jacket potato **P** with following fillings:
  > Baked beans **G**
  > Soft cheese **B**
  > Bolognese-type sauce **B** if meat, with added veg **G**
  > Tuna **B** mixed with a little oil or with salad cream (not mayonnaise)
- Wholewheat crispbreads **P** with following toppings and salad:
  > Soft cheese **B**
  > Tuna or salmon **B**
- Salad made with the following:
  > Dark green salad leaves; chopped, raw peppers; carrots; courgettes; broccoli; corn; beetroot and any other uncooked vegetables; plus sprouts or sprouting beans – *all* **G**. Sprinkle with lightly cracked seeds and/or fresh nuts, e.g. walnuts **B**
  > Hummus/cheese/lean meat **B**
  > Dressing: Udo's Oil or extra-virgin olive oil whisked with balsamic or white wine vinegar, mustard powder, a sprinkle of 'season all' spice (or other herbs or spices),

and a dash of lemon or lime juice. Adjust the ingredients to get a taste you like.

Dinner

- Chilli made with minced meat **B** (or Quorn mince **B**/**G**) plus vegetables and beans **G**. Serve with brown basmati rice **P** and a dark green mixed salad **G**.

- Curry made with meat **B** and vegetables **G**, or vegetables **G** and lentils or beans **B**. Serve with basmati rice or a chapati **P** plus plain yoghurt **B** with mint.

- Shepherd's pie made with minced meat **B** (or Quorn mince **B**/**G**) and chopped vegetables **G** topped with sweet potato mash **P**. Serve with extra vegetables **G**.

- Fish pie made with a selection of fish **B** and cooked in white wine and leek sauce with a spoonful of light soft cheese **B**. Top with sweet potato mash **P** and serve with extra vegetables **G**.

- Stir-fry of mixed vegetables **G** with chicken or beef **B**. Serve with quinoa, or rice **P** and salad **G**.

- Salad – see lunch suggestions.

Recipes

This is not a diet, so I encourage you to adapt the dishes and meals you currently cook using the colour-code system as a guide.

Many thanks to Gerry Sweeney, chef at the Amberley Inn, Gloucestershire, for the great colour-code system recipes and top tips!

Chicken and Crème Fraîche with Apples and Mushrooms

Serves 4

30ml (2 tbsp) vegetable oil

60g (2oz) butter

2 onions, finely chopped

4 chicken breasts

400ml (14fl oz) dry cider

400g (14oz) mushrooms, sliced

400ml (14fl oz) low-fat crème fraîche

100g (3½oz) apple purée

1. Heat the oil and half the butter in a saucepan. Add the onions and chicken breasts and brown all over.

2. Add the cider to the pan and simmer for a few minutes.

3. In a separate pan, fry the mushrooms with the rest of the butter until brown. Drain and then add to the chicken and onions and season. Cook on a low heat for 30 minutes.

4. Add the crème fraîche and apple purée to the pan and cook for a further 10 minutes.

5. Serve in a warmed bowl with pasta or new potatoes.

Country Vegetable Soup

Serves 4

50g (1½oz) dried haricot beans

30ml (2 tbsp) vegetable oil

50g (1½oz) fine beans

100g (3½oz) broad beans

100g (3½oz) leeks, finely shredded

100g (3½oz) carrots, diced

100g (3½oz) turnip or swede, diced

100g (3½oz) courgettes

4 tomatoes, deseeded and chopped

50g (1½oz) tomato purée

50g (1½oz) macaroni

1.5 litres (2½ pints) vegetable stock

1. Soak the haricot beans overnight in cold water.

2. Place the fine and broad beans in a pot of cold water, bring to the boil and gently simmer for 20 minutes. Remove from the heat and run under cold running water.

3. In a separate pan, heat the oil. Add the leeks and sweat for 3 minutes.

4. Add the carrots and turnip or swede and cook for a further 2 minutes.

5. Add the haricot beans, cover with the vegetable stock. Add all other ingredients and cook until tender.

6. Season and serve.

Chef's tip: Liquidize 50g (1½oz) of basil, one garlic clove and 15ml (1 tbsp) of olive oil. Swirl on top of your soup as a garnish.

Tofu Pâté with Green Peppercorn and Paprika Sauce

Serves 4

For the pâté

300g (10oz) tofu

100g (3½oz) sunflower seeds

100ml (3fl oz) low-fat crème fraîche

1 carrot, finely grated

25g (1oz) chives, finely chopped

1. Liquidize the tofu, sunflower seeds and crème fraîche, and season.

2. Put mixture in a bowl and add the carrot and chives.

3. Place in the fridge until chilled.

For the sauce

>   400g (14oz) can of plum tomatoes
>
>   25g (1oz) crushed green peppercorns
>
>   12g (half a tbsp) paprika
>
>   12ml (2 tsp) sunflower oil
>
>   200ml (6fl oz) low-fat crème fraîche
>
>   Juice of half a lemon

1. Purée the tomatoes, peppercorns and paprika with a hand blender.

2. Pour the oil into a pan and then heat the mixture gently for
    5 minutes.

3. Add the crème fraîche and bring to the boil.

4. Add the lemon juice and then pass the sauce through a strainer.

5. Serve cool or chilled with the pâté.

Chef's tip: Serve with sweet potato wedges as a main course, or with crudités as a starter – try peppers, carrot batons or celery sticks.

Salmon Stir-fry with Thai Spices

Serves 4

>   Splash of vegetable oil
>
>   4 × 160g (6oz) salmon fillets
>
>   60g (2oz) bean shoots
>
>   15g (half a tbsp) ginger, grated
>
>   30g (1oz) carrots, finely sliced
>
>   30g (1oz) celery, finely sliced
>
>   30g (1oz) courgettes, finely sliced
>
>   1 red chilli, deseeded and finely chopped

Lemon grass – half a stalk

50g (1½oz) coriander, chopped

15ml (1 tbsp) fish stock

15ml (1 tbsp) soy sauce

30g (2 tbsp) toasted sesame seeds

1. In a frying pan or wok, fry the salmon with a small amount of vegetable oil for a couple of minutes each side. Remove from the pan and keep warm.

2. In the same pan or wok, stir-fry the bean shoots, ginger and vegetables for a few minutes. Add the chilli and lemon grass and cook for 5 minutes.

3. Add the fish stock and soy sauce.

4. Add the coriander and put the stir-fry mixture into four warmed bowls.

5. Place the warm salmon fillet on top of the vegetables and sprinkle with the toasted sesame seeds.

Plaice Fillet with Mushrooms and Pak Choi

Serves 4

Vegetable oil for shallow frying

300g (10oz) plaice, cut into goujons

30ml (2 tbsp) soy sauce

10g (2 tsp) fresh ginger, grated

10g (2 tsp) cornflour

1 egg white, lightly beaten

50g (1½oz) mushrooms, sliced

1 onion, finely chopped

2 cloves of garlic, crushed

2 small pak choi – leaves separated

40ml (1½fl oz) fish or chicken stock

1.   Put the plaice goujons in a small bowl. Add half the soy sauce, half the ginger and half the cornflour and stir to combine.

2.   Add the egg white, season with salt and pepper and stir again.

3.   Remove the goujons from the mixture and shallow fry in vegetable oil in a frying pan or wok until golden brown. Drain on a piece of kitchen roll.

4.   Heat a little more oil in the pan or wok. Add the mushrooms, onions and garlic and fry for 1 minute.

5.   Add the pak choi leaves, stir-fry for 1–2 minutes, or until they have wilted slightly.

6.   Blend the remaining cornflour, ginger and soy sauce with the stock in a small jug. Pour into the pan/wok and stir-fry for 1–2 minutes.

7.   Place the goujons into a serving dish and pour over the mushroom and pak choi sauce.

Chickpea Curry

Serves 4

Splash of vegetable oil

3 carrots, diced

3 celery stalks, diced

1 leek, roughly chopped

2 onions, roughly chopped

2 fresh chillies, finely chopped

50g (2 tbsp) curry powder

250ml (8fl oz) vegetable stock (reduce or add more, depending on desired consistency)

2 × 400g (14oz) tins chopped tomatoes

2 gloves garlic, minced

100g (4 tbsp) tomato purée

Pinch of turmeric

2 × 400g (14oz) tins chickpeas

1. Heat the oil in a saucepan. Add all the vegetables, plus the onions, chillies and curry powder. Cook on a low heat for 1 minute.

2. Add three-quarters of the vegetable stock, the tomatoes, garlic, tomato purée and turmeric.

3. Bring to the boil and simmer for 10 minutes.

4. With a hand blender, liquidize to a fine sauce, adding the remaining stock (or additional stock) as needed. Cook for a further 10 minutes on a medium heat.

5. Add the chickpeas and cook for a further 5 minutes.

6. Serve in warmed bowls with boiled rice.

Healthy Quick-start Two-week Plan

For the first two weeks of using the colour-code system, if you follow the Healthy Quick Start programme I'm about to give you, it will take the stress off your liver and other systems. This way, your body can establish a level of health that will enable you to burn more fat, more effectively – and you know from the earlier chapters how beneficial this will be. You may or may not lose a significant amount of weight over this two-week period (although many people do experience a significant drop in weight, especially if they are prone to bloating and fluid retention). The goal is to establish for you a healthy physiology that will enable you to lose more weight in the medium and longer term, so it is well worth the effort.

The Healthy Quick Start is not a strict detox – and it isn't that different from the previous general recommendations in this chapter – but it is a more disciplined way of eating and using the same principles, to give your body a boost and maximize your future progress. Although there are recommendations within the colour-code system as to what to eat, the Healthy Quick Start is more about *what not to eat for two weeks.*

As mentioned in Chapter 13, this is purely optional. If it looks too hard or you see it as a traditional diet, **do not do it**. Only follow it if you can see it fitting in with your lifestyle and you won't feel deprived. Of course, you can come back and do it anytime to give yourself a boost further down the line if you choose to.

Healthy Quick-Start General Guidelines

Overall the Healthy Quick Start Plan has a higher percentage of **G**, high quality, low fat **B** and minimal **P**. It excludes all processed or refined high-sugar foods, alcohol and caffeine.

- Aim to have at least one raw, vegetable-based meal (can be served with lightly cooked lean meat or fish) per day. This is likely to be in the form of salad. Have unlimited amounts of raw or lightly cooked vegetables, but aim for a minimum of three portions per day. This may be as salads or chopped veg to dip into homemade guacamole or hummus.

- Try raw or lightly cooked cauliflower rice. Place cauliflower florets in a blender for just a few seconds (too long and it will go to mush). This can be served as raw rice, or very lightly stir-fried in a tiny bit of vegetable oil and a splash of water. Works well as an alternative to couscous, which is wheat based.

- Limit the amount of red meat, or ideally exclude it altogether for two weeks, in favour of lightly cooked fish or white meat.

- Have a handful of fresh nuts and seeds every day, and use unrefined extra-virgin olive or Udo's Oil (*see supplements, page 268*) for salad dressings.

- Meat – have at least two meat-free days a week, and if practical or possible, buy organic. If using red meat, cook it rare or medium rare as this is easier to digest.

- Fish – eat oily fish (not farmed) at least twice a week.

- Dairy – choose organic milk and cheese if practical or possible. Avoid hard cheese in favour of soft cheese and have a maximum of two portions of dairy per day – for example, one portion of milk in cereal and one portion of cheese in a salad or meal.

- Drink plenty of water in addition to the drinks suggested, so you can flush out toxins.

- Consume lots of high-fibre foods (you'll automatically be doing this because you'll be eating raw and lightly cooked vegetables) as this will aid the clearing process.

- Aim to eat a minimum of three portions of raw vegetables per day, either in salads or chopped as snacks.

- Add as many cruciferous (leafy) vegetables to your meals as possible. Boil them in a little water or steam them.

- Eat foods that contain EFAs, such as olives, avocados, uncooked nuts and seeds (broken to release the oils), fish (raw sushi fish, without the rice, is ideal). Or use Udo's Oil (*see supplements, page 268*).

- Eat three times per day or more – do not skip meals because you need to maintain a constant blood sugar to avoid stressing the liver.

- Avoid bread (absolutely no white bread) and all wheat products whenever possible.

- Use quinoa instead of rice, potatoes (except sweet potatoes, which are fine) and pasta.

While you are on the plan, it is important to avoid the following:

- Alcohol
- Caffeine
- Tobacco
- Foods from the **R** group
- Processed and packaged foods
- Wheat (whenever possible).

Support for Your Liver

You will find stopping caffeine a lot easier if you cut down gradually over a week; if you are a caffeine craver, stopping it straight off will result in you having headaches and feeling rough for three to five days. This runs counter to everything you can achieve on this programme – I want you to feel good and build positive anchors, not negative ones – so stop caffeine at your own pace and gradually replace it with herbal or fruit teas. Here's a list of some liver-cleansing herbs and foods that are available as teas, drinks or supplements from your health shop. They can also all be blended together to make a juice that will support and cleanse the liver:

- Milk thistle
- Dandelion
- Artichoke leaves
- Pomegranate (not processed)
- Beetroot (not pickled)
- Grapefruit

- Berries
- Rosemary
- Liquorice.

Sample Meals for the Healthy Starter Plan

Breakfast

- Take a large cup or a small mug of frozen (or fresh, if in season) berries and blend them with an organic yoghurt in a simple hand blender.
- Homemade juice using beetroot, cabbage, apples, celery or similar fruit and vegetables.
- Organic, sugar-free muesli with chopped apples.
- Organic eggs scrambled or poached.
- SynerProTein drink (see *supplements section, page 268*).

Lunch

- Homemade vegetable soup with any vegetables of your choice and include lentils, beans or pulses to increase the protein element and make it more satisfying.
- Salad (including chopped or grated raw vegetables) with fish or lean meat and homemade salad dressing (e.g. extra-virgin olive oil, or Udo's Oil with balsamic vinegar, mustard powder and a light squeeze of lemon or lime).

Dinner

- Salad with a **B** component (as above).
- Stir-fry of crispy vegetables (lightly cooked in oil) with garlic, ginger, fresh chillies, etc. (add other spices to taste), with

lightly cooked fish or meat. Serve with quinoa.

- Lentil and vegetable bake or casserole served with leafy green vegetables.

Snacks

- Raw vegetables and hummus (homemade by crushing chickpeas with low-fat crème fraîche and flavourings of your choice e.g. garlic, chilli etc.).
- Apples and other crunchy fruit.
- Homemade berry smoothies.
- Fresh, uncooked nuts and seeds (crack the husks to release the oil).

Drinks

- Fruit teas, green tea, white tea, hot or cold water with lemon slices, any diluted, unsweetened fruit juice.
- After the first two weeks are over, you can begin to adapt the system to suit your own likes and dislikes; don't eat something just because it's healthy – whatever nutrient it contains can almost certainly be found in something else. I wanted to 'train' myself to like green and white tea, so every time I tasted them I closed my eyes and thought of a taste I really enjoyed, and anchored it to the taste of the green and white tea. After a few attempts it worked well and I drink these teas every day. However, for some reason my taste buds just will not accept the taste of olives, no matter what I try and anchor it to! So I use unrefined olive oil and make sure I get plenty of EFAs from other sources. Although food is medicine, it shouldn't taste like medicine!

Exercise

During the two weeks of the healthy starter plan, aim to be active, but not aggressive, with your exercise regime. If you are a non-exerciser, aim to walk briskly or swim for at least 20–30 minutes at least four times a week (or a little less if this is too much for you). If you are already a regular exerciser then be sure to maintain your usual level, but don't increase it during these two weeks. Remember: the aim of the plan is to get healthy! Part of that process is to allow your body to rest and recover and enable the nutrients you are taking in to work to best effect. Once your body has done that, it will respond much better when you introduce some new and more challenging activities, especially those that increase muscle tone (LBM) such as resistance training – which may be going to a gym or just cycling or walking up hills instead of staying on the flat!

Supplements

A question I get asked all the time is, 'Which supplements help weight loss?' You can be forgiven for thinking that a pill or a potion may help because you are constantly being bombarded with advertisements for this or that formula that purports to 'aid weight loss'. The truth is that the best supplements are the ones that promote overall health rather than weight loss – the healthier you are, the easier it is to burn fat.

While making it clear that 'supplement' means *as well as*, not *instead of*, I would recommend the following supplements (some of which I take myself):

- **Healthy Starter Pack**: A herbal mix to cleanse the liver and other organs and promote bowel health. Visit www. powertochange.me.uk and click on 'Nature's Sunshine'.

(found at the bottom of the homepage). This is a supplement that I recommend to most of my weight-loss clients as it does help cleanse the liver and give your digestive system a boost.

- **Super Supplemental Vitamins & Minerals**: Visit www. powertochange.me.uk and click on the 'Nature's Sunshine' link on the home page. These can be ordered online and delivered direct to your door.

- **Udo's Oil**: This can be used as a supplement or drizzled on salads (I stir mine into some yoghurt and then pour it on my cereal), or added to stir-fries after cooking. Available direct to your door from www.udoschoice.co.uk.

- **SynerProTein drink**: A blend of natural amino acids with the right balance of carbohydrates, this can be used as an occasional meal replacement, or regularly as a breakfast drink. Visit www.powertochange.me.uk and click on the 'Nature's Sunshine' link on the home page and they can be delivered direct to your door.

· ·

Chapter 16

Setting Your Goal

A t the beginning of the book I told you that the goal setting exercise was at the end. Take a moment to think about what you want to achieve on this programme. What is your desired outcome? Is it really just to lose weight, or is to feel different about yourself? Perhaps you want to feel in control or more confident? What is it that you think losing weight will bring you? What do you really want? And why?

I often think the word 'goal' is misunderstood in this context. The goal is what you want to achieve, but it is based *entirely* on what you *do*. So, if you make your goal relate to your behaviours, then you will automatically achieve the outcome you want. For example, if you only eat junk food and you want to be size 12, you make your goal not to eat junk food – replacing it with planned cooked meals and snacks. You will then automatically lose weight and reach your desired size 12. When you make the *behaviours* the goal, the weight takes care of itself.

A critical factor in achieving a goal is to be *really clear* about what you want to achieve. To do this you need to write it down, and then create an action plan using tried-and-tested principles in order to achieve it. Have a look back at Napoleon Hill's

14 principles (*see page 42*). This book has been designed to guide you through these, and if you have completed all the exercises and 'played full-out', then you are well on the way. The final step is to plan your strategy, which you've no doubt been forming as you've read the book. If you are following the Placebo Diet at Home programme, you will be guided you through a process, but if you are just reading this book then we will do it another way:

Creating a Strategy

Step 1: What dress/trouser size do you want to achieve?

I want to be size ....

Approximately how much weight do you want to lose (to the nearest 2–2.5kg or 4–5lbs)?

I want to lose ....

The reason I have put size first and not weight, is because weight does not take into account body composition. For example, someone like Arnold Schwarzenegger might weigh the same as a sumo wrestler, and both would be classified as 'morbidly obese', but clearly one is fat and the other muscular, so body composition is key. Size is a guide and must be taken in context with shape.

Step 2: When do you want to achieve it by?

I want to be size .... by ....

Make sure your desired size and the time frame you have given are realistic. As a guide, you can lose approximately one dress size per month or up to 3kg (7lbs) if you go from a starting point of unhealthy eating and inactivity to healthy eating and activity. If your time frame expects a loss of more than one dress size per month, you may need to rethink it, as it's important you know it's genuinely achievable.

On a scale of 1–10, if one is none and 10 is full-out commitment, how much effort are you prepared to put in, starting today? Be honest. You can still get results at 5/10, but of course it will take longer because you are not really embracing the changes wholeheartedly and are more likely to slip back into your old ways. In my own case I would give myself 8½/10 in terms of the amount of time I devote to healthy eating and activity. I still go out for a slap-up meal sometimes and I don't believe a 'holier than thou' approach works very well for most people. If it's too strict it becomes a diet, and it's unpleasant, so for all the reasons you have learnt in this book, you are likely to self-sabotage. For real success you need to be 8 or above on this programme, but you don't need to be perfect. For the exercise below you will need to refer back to some of the exercises in the book. Now that you have a good understanding of how your body works and what to eat, you will find your unconscious mind is filling up with ideas about how to combine the behavioural techniques with the colour-code system in a way that suits you.

Exercise

Get six pieces of A4 paper or card and write the following on them:

- 1 day
- 1 week
- 1 month
- 3 months
- 6 months
- 12 months

Look at the cards and, based on your desired outcome and time frame, make a note of the point at which you will have achieved your new dress size. If it's longer than 12 months, simply add a seventh card.

Now, refer back to the exercises in the earlier chapters of the book and in your journal and note all the things you want or need to change. Which of these changes can you commit to doing *within the next 24 hours* in order to make a positive difference in the way you think and behave? Write them on the first piece of paper or card; aim to write at least two things and make sure one is a psychological change (for example, 'Stop telling myself I'm useless and start giving myself positive encouragement') and the other a nutritional change (for example, 'Stop snacking on crisps and get some fresh nuts and seeds or fruit instead').

After you have read the whole of this instruction, place the first piece of paper or card on the floor and stand behind it. Take a deep breath and step onto it. As you do so, imagine the changes you have written down are being uploaded into your mind. Imagine this is *really* happening, and as you do, create in your mind's eye images of you *doing* these things the next day. When you have done this fully, step off the paper or card and imagine that day has already happened, and that you already have a day's experience under your belt.

On the second piece of paper or card, write down what you want to change over the next seven days (in addition to the changes you have already made or implemented on the first day). As before, make sure you include psychological and nutritional changes. In the same way as before, place the paper or card on the floor and stand behind it. Take a deep breath and step onto it, and as you do this, imagine these changes are being uploaded into your mind. Imagine this is really happening and as you do, create in your mind's eye images of you doing these things over the next seven days. When you have done this fully, step off and imagine the week has already happened, and that now you have a week's experience under your belt.

When you have fully done this, you really can see a week's worth of events having happened (which may highlight some pitfalls as well as benefits).

Repeat the exercise in exactly the same way for one month, three months and so on until you have a clear strategy on all six cards, *and* you have literally walked through and experienced it becoming reality.

Now lay all the cards in a row in front of you like stepping stones. After reading this instruction fully, step on to the first card and relive that first day again. Then move straight on to the first week and relive that again, then the first month and so on. When you get to your last card, and you have changed all the things you need to change to achieve your goal, turn around and look back at how far you have come. See the old 'you' standing way back, and send 'you' the wisdom you have now from *experiencing* these 12 months of change. Talk to 'you' out loud, tell 'you' not to worry and that 'you' can do it because you already have! Tell 'you' that as soon as 'you' change your mind, your body will start to change. Not at the same rate, but it will change definitely and purposefully into the healthy new shape you are now, in the future. As you look back at all the changes you have made, do you like what you see?

Close your eyes, and create a powerful, positive anchor for this feeling of certainty and achievement (*see page 116*). Create absolute *faith* in your ability to achieve this, because you already have made the changes you wanted to make. Did you see those changes?

You may wish to squeeze your fist at this point, or press your tongue against the roof of your mouth (this is often used to aid focus). Or you can create your own physical movement that you can repeat anywhere, and at any time.

• •

These six pieces of paper or card are now your strategy. You now have everything you need. But like all the best strategies, they are flexible. They can be improved and changed as you continue to develop new skills, and as positive thoughts become second nature. I recommend that you take a few minutes to lay the cards out and repeat this walk through *at least* once per week. The more you repeat it (with full-on emotion), the more entrenched it will become in your unconscious and your new neurological maps will become stronger and stronger. Imagination is your reality. When you change in your mind, your body will change, too.

I wish you joy for your journey. The best way to learn is to teach. Now you know the secret, share it by doing it yourself and teaching others who also want to change. You have the power to passively teach by example, without even speaking a word (through mirror neurons), and inspire others around you in a way that is more powerful than words.

....

Recommended Reading

Some of the authors who have inspired me with their beautiful books, and whom I would like to thank and recommend are:

Richard Bach – for everything he has ever written! Especially *Jonathan Livingston Seagull* (Turnstone Press, 1972) and *Hypnotizing Maria* (Hampton Roads Publishing, 2009)

Dr Joe Dispenza for *You Are the Placebo* (Hay House, 2014)

Charles Duhigg for *The Power Of Habit* (Random House Books, 2013)

Udo Erasmus for *Fats That Heal, Fats That Kill* (Alive Books, 1993)

David R. Hamilton for *Why Kindness is Good For You* (Hay House, 2010)

Louise Hay for *You Can Heal Your Life* (Hay House, 2004)

Daniel Kahneman for *Thinking, Fast and Slow* (Penguin, 2012)

Bruce Lipton for *The Biology Of Belief* (Hay House, 2011, 2015)

Michael A. Singer for *The Untethered Soul* (New Harbinger Publications, 2007)

Index

ABOUT THE AUTHOR

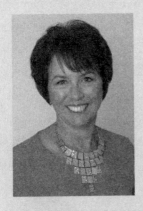

Janet Thomson is an outstanding life coach with a unique blend of skills and experience. She holds a Masters degree in Nutrition & Exercise Science, is an NLP (Neuro-Linguistic Programming) Master Practitioner and Trainer, a TFT (Thought Field Therapy) Diagnostic Therapist and a registered Clinical Hypnotherapist. She combines these advanced skills with over 20 years of experience working with clients on an individual basis and in groups and seminars. This has firmly established her as a leader in the field of Personal Development and Achievement.

Janet became a bestselling author with her first book and fitness video, *Fat to Flat*. She has appeared on GMTV and BBC1, and was resident Health & Fitness Expert and Life Coach for ITV Central. Janet regularly delivers seminars for both the general public and other instructors, and she coaches in the UK and abroad. Most recently she took her inspirational programmes to Dar Al-Hekma University in Saudi Arabia, where she taught her 'Change Your Mind' programme to over 400 students and faculty members.

Having previously owned and run three health clubs in the Midlands, Janet now runs her own Power To Change private coaching and consultancy practice, and is part of Growing Wellness, a company dedicated to improving the emotional health of staff in large companies. Those lucky enough to work with Janet enjoy great results and lasting change, making her one of the most sought-after coaches in the UK.

www.theplacebodiet.co.uk
www.powertochange.me.uk

Notes

Notes

HAY HOUSE

Look within

Join the conversation about latest products,
events, exclusive offers and more.

 Hay House UK

 @HayHouseUK

 @hayhouseuk

♥ healyourlife.com

We'd love to hear from you!